ASSESSMENT OF BRAIN DAMAGE

WILEY SERIES ON PERSONALITY PROCESSES

IRVING B. WEINER, *Editor*
Case Western Reserve University

INTERACTION IN FAMILIES
by Elliot G. Mishler and Nancy E. Waxler

SOCIAL STATUS AND PSYCHOLOGICAL DISORDER: A Causal Inquiry
by Bruce P. Dohrenwend and Barbara Dohrenwend

PSYCHOLOGICAL DISTURBANCE IN ADOLESCENCE
by Irving B. Weiner

ASSESSMENT OF BRAIN DAMAGE: A Neuropsychological Key Approach
by Elbert W. Russell, Charles Neuringer, and Gerald Goldstein

BLACK AND WHITE IDENTITY FORMATION
by Stuart Hauser

THE HUMANIZATION PROCESSES: A Social, Behavioral Analysis of Children's Problems
by Robert L. Hamblin, David Buckholdt, Daniel Ferritor, Martin Kozloff, and Lois Blackwell

ADOLESCENT SUICIDE
by Jerry Jacobs

TOWARD THE INTEGRATION OF PSYCHOTHERAPY
by John M. Reisman

MINIMAL BRAIN DYSFUNCTION IN CHILDREN
by Paul Wender

LSD: PERSONALITY AND EXPERIENCE
by Harriet Linton Barr, Robert J. Langs, Robert R. Holt, Leo Goldberger, and George S. Klein

TREATMENT OF THE BORDERLINE ADOLESCENT: A Developmental Approach
by James F. Masterson

PSYCHOPATHOLOGY: Contributions from the Biological, Behavioral, and Social Sciences
edited by Muriel Hammer, Kurt Salzinger, and Samuel Sutton

ABNORMAL CHILDREN AND YOUTH: Therapy and Research
by Anthony Davids

ASSESSMENT OF BRAIN DAMAGE

A Neuropsychological Key Approach

ELBERT W. RUSSELL

Veterans Administration Hospital
Cincinnati, Ohio

CHARLES NEURINGER

University of Kansas

GERALD GOLDSTEIN

Veterans Administration Hospital
Topeka, Kansas

with the assistance of Carolyn H. Shelly

WILEY-INTERSCIENCE
A Division of John Wiley & Sons, Inc.
New York · London · Sydney · Toronto

10 9 8 7 6 5 4 3

Library of Congress Catalogue Card Number: 73-121914

ISBN 0-471-74550-2

Printed in the United States of America

To the memory of Martin Scheerer

Preface

The study of brain damage in this book is a product of several years of research, carried out in the neuropsychology laboratory at the Topeka Veterans Administration Hospital. The procedures used in this laboratory are primarily those developed by the late Ward C. Halstead and later expanded by Ralph M. Reitan, Hallgrim Kløve, Homer B. C. Reed, James Reed, and other associates of Dr. Reitan. The book is intended for the clinician and psychology student who uses the Halstead Battery or who wishes to learn about its use. Its major aim is to demonstrate that the neuropsychological laboratory, as first conceptualized by Halstead, can make a substantial contribution to our understanding of brain-behavior relationships in human beings. We also show that such a laboratory in a clinical setting can provide useful and valid procedures for evaluating patients with brain lesions.

We should like to express our appreciation to several individuals who were helpful in producing this book. Special appreciation is expressed to Dr. Phillip M. Rennick who worked extensively with us in the initial stages of the research program. Dr. Rennick devised the rating system we employed and kindly gave us his permission to use it in our research. He also suggested several of the hypotheses that were later incorporated into the keys. Dr. D. Bernard Foster of the Menninger Foundation was most helpful in providing neurological documentation. Without his assistance and the cooperation of the Neurology Service at the Topeka Veterans Administration Hospital this research could not have been accomplished. Indebtedness is expressed to the late James K. Majors who did most of the clerical work involved in running the keys. The cooperation of the Research Committee of the Topeka Veterans Administration Hospital is also acknowledged. In addition, we wish to acknowledge the assistance of the Computation Center at the University of Kansas, where most of the data analysis and development of the computer program for the keys were done. The contribution of Mrs. Carolyn H. Shelly went far beyond writing the computer programs, for she did a great deal of the data analysis and was of great help in proofreading the manuscript. Finally, we should like to acknowledge the work of Dr. Irving B. Weiner, the series editor, for his many valuable suggestions and extensive editorial comments.

ELBERT W. RUSSELL
CHARLES NEURINGER
GERALD GOLDSTEIN

Lawrence, Kansas
January 1970

Contents

ASSESSMENT OF BRAIN DAMAGE

CHAPTER 1

Introduction

In recent years the battery of psychological tests for brain damage, developed by Halstead (1947) and later modified by Reitan (1955b), has received increasing use for the diagnosing of brain damage. Reitan (1964a) has demonstrated that this battery can identify etiology and locale of brain lesions with a high degree of accuracy. He also found that such diagnoses can be made more accurately using "clinical intuition" than through the use of statistical methods. Using only test results from the Halstead Battery, Reitan succeeded in correctly identifying localization and etiology of brain damage at levels of accuracy far exceeding chance, through the use of an "intuitive" method (chi-square significance was beyond the .001 level). Then he subjected the same test data to an analysis of variance, and only a few significant differences were found. These few differences would not have enabled one to differentiate the brain damaged from the nonbrain damaged groups as well as when using the clinical inference method. Reitan summarized his results as follows: "The outstanding finding of Study 2 (which used statistics) must be viewed as the paucity of significant differences between the groups compared" (Reitan, 1964a, p. 311). "Certainly more sophisticated statistical techniques than were used in this study could have been applied, but if the orientation were directed to differences in intergroup mean levels, we suspect that the analysis still would not do justice to the data. . . . unknown or uncontrolled factors apparently operate to 'wash out' the differences that appear to exist between lesions varying in type and location when conventional methods of analysis are applied to the data . . ." (p. 312).

Although this study revealed that clinical intuition was superior to statistical methods, it also posed the problem of objectifying clinical inference; that is, as Reitan stated, ". . . the necessary information for the inferences was present in the data . . ." (Reitan, 1964a, p. 312). Thus a significant problem in brain damage research is that of finding an objective method of duplicating the results of the inferential technique.

Since Reitan has apparently demonstrated the limitations inherent in traditional statistical methods, another kind of objective method would appear to be required. One such method has been used in biology for almost three centuries. It is the Taxonomic Key. If we examine the verbalized inferences made by neuropsychologists such as Reitan, we will find that such inferences often resemble the keying method in their logical form. The keying method is used by biologists to identify a species which they have collected. It is not a means of classifying a species (Sokal & Sneath, 1963) but rather a means of determining the class into which a particular case or species fits. It is essentially a diagnostic method, a way of locating a species within the framework of a preexisting, established taxonomic system.

As an objective method, the keying technique represents a type of reasoning by elimination. A Biological Key using objective and rather unvarying characteristics of organisms gradually subdivides the total group of organisms into increasingly smaller groups (kingdom, order, family, etc.) until the species has been defined. This method of reasoning by elimination can be seen in the inferential processes used by neuropsychologists to determine type and location of brain damage. Although the inference process may not follow this form in all instances, it does appear to represent a prototype for much of the thinking used in classification of cases. It offers an approach to objective resolution of diagnostic difficulties that would appear to be more adequate than those that have made use of conventional statistical methods. Several authors in recent years have suggested similar methods (Haynes & Sells, 1963; Wechsler, 1958, p. 167). Wechsler calls his technique of diagnosis the *method of successive sieves,* a method in which a series of test patterns is sequentially applied to the same population.

To build such a Key for brain damage it becomes immediately obvious that the keying method as used in biology would need extensive modification. A major obstacle in translating the biological keying method into a Key for diagnosing brain damage is that brain damage is much more variable in its characteristics than are biological species. As fully discussed later, however, other considerations make such a Key possible. In order to test the feasibility of a brain damage Key, a preliminary Key incorporating modifications of the Biological Key was constructed and tried out in a pilot study. The results were quite encouraging in that they suggested that a Key could be constructed to categorize cases into (a) not brain damaged, (b) right hemisphere, (c) left hemisphere, and (d) diffuse brain damage groups. The present study represents a further attempt to test the feasibility of such a Key with a large number of cases. Two Keys, one for lateralization of brain damage and one for several major process categories of brain damage, such as acute and static, were constructed and evaluated.

The present report consists of a description of the development of two

Neuropsychological Keys based on verbalized rules of inference used by neuropsychologists, application of these Keys to a population of brain damaged and nonbrain damaged patients, and an evaluation of how accurately these Keys predict the neurological diagnosis. A second aspect of the research involved an evaluation of the extent to which the predictions made by the Keys matched those made by a neuropsychologist using the clinical inference method. By making this dual comparison the reader may be informed of the level of accuracy of the Key method in predicting against a neurological criterion, as well as of the extent to which the Keys agree with the clinician in predicting neurological deficit from psychological test results. Since the Keys are based on the Reitan modification of the Halstead Neuropsychological Battery, the following two chapters trace the history of this battery and outline its underlying rationale. Historical material concerning biological keys and their application to psychology are also included in these chapters.

CHAPTER 2

The Halstead Neuropsychological Battery and Its Modifications by Reitan

The development of the Halstead Battery and its modifications, along with the approach to the investigation of brain damage associated with the battery, have an organic quality. Even in Halstead's original work this flux and active experimentation could be observed in the changes that were made in selecting the tests for the battery. This process has continued in its subsequent development.

ESTABLISHMENT OF HALSTEAD'S LABORATORY

Halstead established the first neuropsychological laboratory for the study of brain-behavior relationships in humans at the University of Chicago in 1935 (Halstead, 1947). Many of the procedures that have since become vital parts of human neuropsychology were begun there. The first and perhaps most important of these was the creation of a close relationship between psychologists and neurosurgeons. Without full cooperation between members of these two disciplines, research in this area is almost impossible.

Subjects were referred to Halstead's laboratory from the University of Chicago Clinics by neurosurgeons Percival Bailey, Paul Bucy, A. Earl Walker and several other medical specialists. "For perhaps the first time in the history of modern neurosurgery, a group of neurologists and neurosurgeons have fully cooperated in making available their cases for careful study by experimental methods," wrote Halstead (1947, p. 31).

Another innovation that can be attributed to Halstead was the use of trained testers who were not professional psychologists. Although at first Halstead administered his own tests, later he trained nonprofessional personnel to do the testing. This innovation allowed for a far more extensive data collection than would have been possible if the tests had only been administered by professional psychologists. This procedure has been continued in most other neuropsychological laboratories and was utilized in the present study.

DEVELOPMENT OF THE CONCEPT OF A BATTERY

The results that emerged from this laboratory were quite fruitful. Halstead developed a battery of psychological tests that was to become the basis for the Reitan modification of the Halstead Neuropsychological Battery. The utilization of a battery of tests was begun before its advantages became clear. Halstead noted in his book, *Brain and Intelligence* (1947), that he developed the battery, originally, not as a better means of studying the effects of brain damage but rather as a means of investigating "biological intelligence."

Halstead was searching for a way to overcome the difficulties that had beset intelligence testing in the late twenties and thirties. "It is apparent that no generally accepted theoretical framework as to the nature of psychometric intelligence has thus far been developed in support of the many measuring devices which are now widely applied. . . . Is X a single or a multiple factor? Is it predominantly environmentally determined, or is it a direct reflector of basic biological functions of the organism?" (Halstead, 1947, pp. 12–13).

What Halstead meant by biological intelligence was not made particularly clear in his book. He attempted to avoid the learning-innateness controversy and feared to call the intelligence he was examining "innate." At a later time Halstead defined biological intelligence as intelligence that was relatively free of cultural considerations and was "general" (Halstead, 1951a, 1951b). He believed that biological intelligence was different from the "psychometric intelligence" measured by the usual intelligence tests. It was more closely related to the human nervous system, and contributed to "man's survival as an organism" (Halstead, 1947, p. 7) and as such it constituted his adaptive capacity.

In attempting to isolate this biological form of intelligence Halstead felt that he could use factor analysis, a technique that had recently come into prominence, on a large group of tests which were related to brain damage. Previous neurological studies appeared to have demonstrated a relationship between brain process and "intelligence" but little in the way of measurement had been attempted, especially on humans (Halstead, 1947, Chap. IV).

In this study, from his original group of 27 tests, he selected 13 tests which yielded objective scores and "which seemed likely to reflect some component of biological intelligence" (Halstead, 1947, p. 39). Of his pool of 237 cases, 50 lobectomies were chosen as his primary subjects. Their lesion, which was produced by an operation, could be fairly precisely located. The rest of the pool consisted of 30 controls, which he attempted to make as heterogeneous as possible—148 head injuries and nine lobotomies.

The battery of 13 tests was applied to the 50 lobectomies and the results were factor analyzed by both Holzinger and Thurstone, yielding four factors each. Thurstone's analysis was reported in the book and became the basis of Halstead's concept of biological intelligence (Halstead, 1947). The various tests that were utilized were also described in this book (Halstead, 1947).

The four factors that Thurstone isolated were designated by Halstead as C, A, P and D. (The matrix for these four factors is given on p. 41 of *Brain and Intelligence,* Halstead, 1947.) Halstead spent a considerable amount of space in his book attempting to determine what these factors were. The factor C was thought to represent a "central integrative field factor" or memory. It loaded on several tests such as the Categories Test, the Henmon-Nelson Test (a verbal IQ test, cf. Halstead, 1947), Speech-Sounds Perception Test and the Halstead Finger-Oscillation Test which is a test of finger tapping speed. The factor A loaded on the Carl Hollow-Square Test (a nonverbal IQ test, cf. Halstead, 1947), the Categories Test and the Tactual Performance Test (Memory). Halstead felt this factor A was an abstraction factor such as Kurt Goldstein had described (Goldstein & Scheerer, 1941). Factor P loaded on the Flicker-Fusion Test, Tactual Performance Test (Memory) and several perceptual tests. Halstead called it a power factor at first, and then later an indication of alertness. The final factor, D, loaded only on the speed measure of the Tactual Performance Test and one perceptual test. It was called a directional or modalities factor having something to do with a person's ability to make use of various other factors in actual expression. These factors were somewhat vague, but include language and various perceptual and motor skills. Shure later attempted to clarify them in a further study with Halstead (Shure & Halstead, 1958). He retained the factor A as an abstraction factor, factor C was related to verbal intelligence and the factor P to vigilance.

By assessing Halstead's four factors on the basis of what has been found since 1947 factors A and C can probably be explained most clearly. The Categories Test, which has been accepted as a test of abstraction, loads on both C and A (though more heavily on A). Thus it cannot alone explain either of them. Among the two IQ tests the nonverbal Carl Hollow-Square Test loads more heavily on A while Henmon-Nelson, a verbal test, loads on C. It appears that Shure was right in thinking that C was a verbal learning factor. One other test does not fit this pattern, however, it is the Finger-Oscillation Test which is a pure and simple motor speed test. It loaded on C, the verbal factor. In Halstead's battery, however, the tapping was recorded for the dominant hand alone, which is usually the right hand. It is now known (Reitan, 1966) that brain damage contralateral to the right hand also affects verbal learning since language abilities are usually mediated by the left side of the brain. On the other hand, nonverbal learning, especially in regard to tasks tapping spatial relations skills, is thought to be primarily related to the right side of the brain (Reitan, 1955a, 1966). Thus it appears that Halstead's C and A factors are primarily measures of laterality. Factor C is a left hemisphere factor and A is a right hemisphere factor. Although this is probably not all they represent, Halstead's factor analysis appears to have discovered a brain-intelligence relationship, though perhaps not the one he thought he had found. It is intriguing to speculate that if Halstead had measured finger tapping on both hands rather than simply on the dominant hand, this relationship would have been clear and he could have realized the differential lateralization of the verbal and nonverbal measures of intelligence several years before Andersen (1950) "discovered" it on the Wechsler-Bellevue.

THE INDEX OF BRAIN DAMAGE

The development of Halstead's impairment index for brain damage was secondary to his search for biological intelligence, yet at this point it appears to have been his most important contribution. In order to demonstrate that the measure of biological intelligence was actually related to brain functions he created the impairment index. He thought that if the index, made up of these factored tests, was affected by brain damage this would constitute good evidence of the validity of these factors or at least of biological intelligence (Halstead, 1947, pp. 105–106). Since he thought that psychometric measures, such as paper and pencil intelligence tests, were not affected by brain damage, especially by frontal damage, the fact that his tests of biological intelligence were affected would demonstrate that his tests were more directly related to brain functioning than psychometric tests.

In his construction of the concept of an index Halstead rejected the procedure that is used to obtain IQ's on psychometric tests which is to average the subtests. He felt that such an index "averages out peaks and troughs of ability and thus obscures these important details" (Halstead, 1947, p. 108). Although the use of a profile could overcome this disadvantage, it did not lend itself to creating a single overall score or index. His solution was to set a cutting point or criterion score for each of the tests that indicated brain damage. When the score on the subtests went over that point, it was counted in the index. Ten tests were used and each contributed one tenth to the index. Thus, if one subject's scores were over the cutting point (or criterion score) on only three of these subtests, his index would be .30.

From his pool of 27 original tests Halstead chose the 10 tests that had the highest *t* value for differentiating brain injury from the normal controls and set a cutting point for each test. By inspection of the profiled difference between his controls and brain damaged subjects he set the index cutting point at .50. If a subject had five test scores in the brain damage range, he was considered to be brain damaged.

The actual tests used were evidently selected from his original pool of 27 tests since they were not entirely the same tests that he used for his factor analysis study. The index used 10 tests, the factor analysis pool used 13 tests and only eight tests were common to both the index and factor analysis pool (Halstead, 1947). Since only the tests that composed the index were used in Reitan's later work, only those tests need to be mentioned. These tests are described by Halstead (1947) and Reitan (1966). They are: Halstead Category Test, Critical Flicker Frequency, Critical Flicker Frequency (Deviation), Tactual Performance Test (Time), Tactual Performance Test (Memory), Tactual Performance Test (Localization), Seashore Rhythm Test, Speech-Sounds Perception Test, Finger Tapping Test, Time-Sense Test (Memory).

The impairment index was found to be quite accurate in predicting the presence of frontal lobe brain damage. Its validity was established through a comparison of test findings with neurological diagnoses. Since these diagnoses were based on neurosurgical evidence, the presence of brain lesions and their approximate locations were unusually well documented. It was found that none of the 30 control cases had a score over .4, and only one of them had a score that high.

Since the publication of Halstead's index it has been discovered that it is not only valid for frontal brain damage but is valid for brain damage in general (Reitan, 1955b, 1956, 1959a, 1959b). Reitan's (1955b) study was specifically designed to validate Halstead's impairment index. A matched pair design was used in which the 50 brain damaged subjects were matched on the basis of color, sex, age and education with 50 normals. The brain damaged subjects had diverse diagnoses and 76% of the controls were hospitalized patients whose medical problems did not involve brain functioning. Among the 50 pairs, not one control had a higher index than his matched partner. Eighty-eight percent had a higher index and 12% had an equal index. The Category Test alone was almost as good as the index itself. It correctly predicted 94% of the brain damaged pairs but 6% of the normal cases had a higher Category score. Recently Shaw (1966) has verified the accuracy of the Category Test in terms of its ability to discriminate between brain damaged and nonbrain damaged individuals.

Reitan's (1955b) analysis of the subtests of the Halstead Battery demonstrated that the Category Test alone was almost as good as the impairment index. Ninety-four percent of the brain damage cases had a poorer Category Test score than prematched controls but 6% had a better score. The rest of the tests in the battery did not do as well, though only the two measures of Critical Flicker Frequency did not give significant results. The result for the Time-Sense Test was significant at the .02 level while the results of the rest of the tests were all over the .001 level of significance.

These results appear to be better than those obtained by almost any other measure of brain damage. The superiority of a battery of tests was also demonstrated as a measure of brain damage. Later studies reviewed by Reitan (1966) have shown that batteries have additional advantages in that they can provide more information about the patient's assets and disabilities, and about the nature of his brain lesion, than can single tests.

Although Halstead's concept of Biological Intelligence has been modified (Reitan, 1956; Shure & Halstead, 1958), his methods (such as the neuropsychological laboratory and the use of a battery of tests, especially the Category Test) and the concept of an index have become integral parts of the many neuropsychological testing programs now in existence.

REITAN'S CONTRIBUTION

Halstead's work was extended by his student, Ralph M. Reitan, who developed more effective approaches to the assessment of brain damage and to brain-behavior relationships. Reitan founded the neuropsychology laboratory at the Indiana University Medical Center with the help of Dr. Robert F. Heimburger, Director of Neurological Surgery, in 1951 (Reitan, 1966). Reitan has described his general program and the results of the program in detail in a chapter in *International Review of Research in Mental Retardation,* N. R. Ellis (Ed.), Vol. I (Reitan, 1966). Consequently only a summary with emphasis on the parts of the program that are directly related to this presentation will be attempted here.

Almost from the beginning the emphasis of Reitan's studies was not directed towards Biological Intelligence. In his concern with the nature of brain functioning his work has generally been closely related to pragmatic neurological problems. In a few studies he attempted to investigate the nature of Biological Intelligence (Reitan, 1956) and in other studies he challenged Kurt Goldstein's theory (Reitan, 1956, 1957, 1958a, 1959b, 1959d) that impairment of abstract reasoning in the damaged brain is a qualitative rather than a quantitative loss.

Much of Reitan's work has involved an exploration of tests to determine their contribution to a battery that could assess the nature of brain damage. His pragmatic approach, however, has often led to the production of information that contributed to more theoretical issues.

The main emphasis of Reitan's work was summarized in his statement that "One of the principal aims of the neuropsychological laboratory has been to effect a meaningful subdivision of the concept of 'brain damage' as such subdivisions relate differentially to psychological measurements" (Reitan, 1966, p. 159). In order to pursue this aim, his program was of necessity exploratory. A large number of data, however, were necessary for such work since specific kinds of brain damage which one might want to study are relatively rare when compared to the total number of brain damage cases. The accumulation of large amounts of data takes a great amount of time. This means that the tests in the battery need to remain relatively constant over a period of time. Thus the selection of tests was of prime importance.

The ability to assess brain damage problems depends on the tests used. Reitan evidently used several guides in his selection of tests (Reitan, 1966). He attempted to sample the major areas of known abilities found in humans. Nonetheless these abilities needed to be related to cerebral lesions in some manner. Since this was an exploratory program, the tests were not based on a particular theoretical framework but were related to those procedures that appeared to be affected by various kinds of brain lesions. Finally there was the hope and growing expectation that this method of psychological assessment of brain damage would be more useful to neurology and psychiatry than previous psychological methods.

Selection of Tests

The first step in selecting tests to explore the nature of cerebral deficit was to validate the procedure of using a battery in general and Halstead's impairment index in particular and to determine whether it tapped most of the functions that might be affected by brain damage. This program laid the foundation for further research.

After this a program of research was initiated to examine the contribution that other tests might make to a battery. A comparison of Halstead's index with the Wechsler-Bellevue Scale, Form I (Wechsler, 1944), demonstrated that "psychometric intelligence" was affected by brain damage as well as "Biological Intelligence" (Reitan, 1959a). Although the index was more sensitive to brain damage, it became apparent that the Wechsler-Bellevue Scale was also affected and could make an important contribution to the battery. Thus it was added to the battery.

It was also found that the Trail Making Test was a valuable instrument in assessment of the effects of brain damage (Armitage, 1946). Studies demonstrated that part B of this test was extremely sensitive to brain damage and differentiated controls from brain damaged patients with only a small overlap (Reitan, 1955c, 1958c) and it was added to the battery.

Other tests added to the battery included a number of techniques derived from the traditional neurological examination (Reitan, 1962). Emphasis was placed on those methods that compared perceptual functioning of the two sides of the body for the purposes of acquiring additional lateralizing information. An aphasia examination is a part of the traditional neurological examination. However, it often does not systematically evaluate the major language skills. An examination that is brief but covers the major functions is the Halstead-Wepman Aphasia Screening Test (Halstead & Wepman, 1949). An abbreviated and slightly modified version of this test was added to the battery. Subsequent research with this test demonstrated that it is sensitive to brain damage (Wheeler & Reitan, 1962) and that it can provide lateralizing information. Several studies (Heimburger & Reitan, 1961; Doehring & Reitan, 1961) demonstrated that the verbal portions of the aphasia test were related in most patients to functioning of the left cerebral hemisphere, whereas the nonverbal or spatial relations parts were related to functioning of the right hemisphere. The most sensitive item in the aphasia test for right hemisphere brain damage was found to be the copying of a Greek cross without lifting the pencil from the paper.

In order to tap the perceptual area of psychological functioning several tests of perceptual functions were constructed which were also modifications of neurological examination procedures. These were the Suppression or Sensory Imperception Test, Finger Agnosia, Finger Tip Writing, and Tactual Form Recognition Tests (Reitan, 1966). These tests compare the perceptual functioning on two sides of the body with each other. As such they usually reflected the laterality of the lesion (Wheeler & Reitan, 1962) when they were affected by brain damage.

Finally the motor element in brain damage was tapped by modifying some of the tests that were already part of the Halstead Battery. The Finger Tapping Test which was limited to the dominant hand in the Halstead Battery was now performed by both hands. Also the Tactual Performance Test scores for dominant and nondominant hand were compared. Clearly significant differences were found that were related to lateralized cerebral damage (Reitan, 1958b).

Two other tests also added to the battery were the Minnesota Multiphasic Personality Inventory (MMPI) and a test for lateral dominance. The MMPI was not used in constructing and evaluating the keys so it will not be discussed. The test for lateral dominance included hand, eye and foot dominance. Since several tests in this battery were based on which hand is dominant, the need for an accurate test of dominance was apparent. These then were the tests that Reitan added to Halstead's original battery.

Aspects of Brain Damage Studied

Utilizing the expanded Halstead Battery described above, Reitan and his collaborators (Reitan, 1966) conducted a series of studies of various aspects of brain damage. These investigations were mostly concerned with the problems of localization, brain damage process and medical diagnosis. The problem of localization involved the ability of the battery, or parts of it, to first lateralize lesions, that is, predict in which hemisphere the lesions are located, and when this had been demonstrated, to determine which quadrant of the brain they affected (Reitan, 1964a). The ability to localize a lesion also required the ability to determine whether or not it was diffuse.

The second kind of investigation dealt with process. Brain lesions tend to change as a function of time and organic processes. This change is now often referred to as brain damage process. When a lesion is traumatic and recent, its effects are usually severe and widespread. It is then considered to be acute. As the lesion becomes older the functional deficit it produces gradually lessens for a period of about two years. Then the effects become stable and the lesion is considered to be static or chronic. The intermediate lesion is a relatively static one. Other types of lesions, such as those produced by tumors, gradually increase in severity and are referred to as progressive lesions. The progressive change in such lesions may occur relatively rapidly or slowly. Congenital brain damage refers to traumatic damage that occurs at or near birth. The effects of such damage may be permanent. Most of Reitan's studies compared acute, relatively static and chronic types of brain damage with each other (Reitan, 1966). In these studies rapidly progressive lesions were considered to be acute, slowly progressive ones were relatively static, and congenital brain damage was placed in the chronic bracket.

Less has been published on the medical diagnosis of types of brain damage, such as open head injury or cerebral arteriosclerosis, though the blind neuropsychological report on the individual cases made by Reitan always contained an attempt to predict the diagnosis of the patient as well as the location of the lesion. The effectiveness of this prediction was usually quite good (Reitan, 1964a). An example of such a report is given at the end of the chapter written for the *International Review of Research in Mental Retardation,* Vol. I (Reitan, 1966).

Two other activities of this laboratory should be mentioned. First, Reitan has been building a neuropsychological test battery for children (Reitan, 1964b). Second, Wheeler has attempted to sharpen the ability of the battery to diagnose types of brain damage by applying a linear discriminant function to the test data. This is a complex method for obtaining optimal weighting of many variables so as to produce a single criterion score for differentiating groups (Wheeler, 1963; Wheeler, Burke & Reitan, 1963; Wheeler & Reitan, 1963). This appears to have been fairly successful but no more successful than the impairment index itself (Wheeler & Reitan, 1963).

RENNICK AND GERALD GOLDSTEIN'S CONTRIBUTION

The brain damage battery used in the present research is a modification of the one used by Reitan. Several changes in it have been made by P. M. Rennick who worked with both Halstead and Reitan. Since most of these changes have not been published, the references in his section are primarily personal communications to the present writers (especially Gerald Goldstein) from Rennick.

Gerald Goldstein developed the neuropsychological battery used in this study in conjunction with Rennick and, to a large extent, adopted Rennick's approach for use at the Topeka Veterans Administration Hospital research facilities.

Reitan began his neuropsychology laboratory using the 10 tests that contributed to Halstead's impairment index. In the study that validated this index (Reitan, 1955b) the two methods of scoring the Critical Flicker Fusion Test were not significant and the Time-Sense Test did not reach the .001 level of significance as did the rest of the tests. This result continued to be evident in the testing program; Rennick eliminated both the Flicker Fusion Test (both scores) and the Time-Sense Test. However, the Trail Making Test and the Digit Symbol Test from the Wechsler Adult Intelligence Scale (WAIS), which had proved quite sensitive to brain damage, were added to the battery.

As has been described, Reitan used the Halstead-Wepman Aphasia Test and several tests of perceptual deficit but these were not quantified as they were usually given. Instead the results were simply described in the examination report. Rennick developed three rating scales for these tests. The verbal parts of the aphasia test had been shown to be sensitive to left-sided damage, whereas the spatial parts, measuring construction apraxia, were sensitive to right-sided damage. Thus a rating scale was made for each of these two parts. Finally a single rating scale was also developed for the perceptual disorder tests. In all three of these rating scales the neuropsychologist examines the raw data and then rates the severity of the deficit based upon his past experience. These three rating scales were added to the total test battery, making twelve scores in all.

Rennick also changed the method of obtaining a total brain damage score. Halstead and Reitan had simply used a single criterion score for each subtest. This was changed so that each test score was placed on a five-point scale, that is, 0 to 4. A score of 1 was normal, 0 was better than average and 2, 3, and 4 represented mild, moderate, and severe impairment, respectively. Except for the three tests rated, numerical norms which transformed the raw scores into the rating point scale were developed for the tests in the battery. Although the scale scores were generally set according to the number of standard deviations from the mean for normal controls, several of the test scaled scores were set on an inferential basis. Generally a score of 1 included the first standard deviation on each side of the mean for normal controls. The standardization population used was a group of patients tested in Reitan's laboratory.

Since all of the tests used in the battery now had a scale score of 0 to 4, Rennick developed an average impairment rating score that could be used in place of Halstead's index. The cutting point for the index was equivalent to the point that separates 1 from 2 on Rennick's scale. All ratings of 2 and above were placed in the brain damaged range. The whole average impairment rating scale could now be used to evaluate not only whether the person had brain damage but also how severe it was. An unpublished statistical analysis found Rennick's Average Impairment Rating scale to be equivalent to the index in determining whether or not the subject has brain damage. Experience with this scaling method has demonstrated that most of the test scaled scores are fairly good indicators of the degree of brain damage. A few of the tests, however, overestimate or underestimate the degree of damage and so they need to have their scale scores reset.

The only major change that G. Goldstein introduced in the battery utilized by this study was the substitution of the WAIS for the Wechsler-Bellevue Test. The complete list of tests used in the present study may be found in Chapter 4.

The tests included five of the original Halstead tests (Categories, Tactual Performance, Speech Perception, Rhythm and Finger Tapping), Reitan's additions (Trail Making, Aphasia Screening, Perceptual Disorders and Lateral Dominance) and the WAIS.

THE BIOLOGICAL KEY

In biology a Key is a method of locating the name of a species in a taxonomic manual. This procedure is not a form of classification but rather it is a means of locating a specimen in a classification system that has already been constructed. Classification consists in grouping species such that their characteristics are consistent with each other. That is, a class or category consists of a group, all of whose members have the same characteristics. A Key uses characteristics of a species to locate the class or category to which the species belongs. Logically it is a form of reasoning by elimination. If a person has a specimen in hand, he can "run" the Key until he locates the name of the specimen by using characteristics of the organism. Keys use objective and rather invariant characteristics of organisms in a systematic manner. They consist of a series of statements about the group of organisms to which the species belong which systematically subdivides the total group into smaller and smaller groups until the desired organism is isolated. Usually the key will use statements to dichotomize a group such as "a) flowers usually solitary"; if the specimen has no solitary flowers, we proceed to the next statement, "b) flowers not solitary." This group of plants without solitary flowers is then further dichotomized until the desired species is reached.

An example of a Key taken from a botany manual (Clements & Clements, 1945) is given below. In this case groups are sometimes divided into more than two parts.

Here is an example used to locate a species within the rose genus.

1. Flowers usually several in a corymb; leaflets mostly 9–11; *R. arkansana*
2. Flowers usually solitary; leaflets mostly 5–7
   a. Stems with 2–3 larger conspicuous spines at base of the leaf stalk
      (1) Flowers 3–5 cm. wide; fruits 7–10 mm. wide; *R. woödsi*
      (2) Flowers 5–8 cm. wide; fruits 12–20 mm. wide, often prickly; *R. nutkána*
   b. Stems very spiny, but without larger conspicuous spines at the base of the leaf stalk; fruit globose to pear-shaped; *R. acicularis*
   (Clements & Clements, 1945, p. 162)

Essentially only two major types of Keys have been used in biology (Voss, 1952), the parallel type and the indented type. The previous example of a Key was the indented type which is most often used in botany. An example of the parallel type, which is more often used in zoology, is the following:

Order Homoptera

134a Antennae below the eye at side of head—Family Fulgoridae
134b Antennae in front of and between the eyes, 135
135a Hind tibia with two rows of spines—Family Cicadellidae
135b Hind tibia with a circlet of spines at apex—Family Cercopidae

Order Orthoptera

136a Legs fitted for leaping—tarsi three or four segmented, 138
136b Legs not fitted for leaping—tarsi five segments, 137
137a Body oval, depressed—Family Blattidae
137b Body elongate, not depressed—Family Mantidae
138a Tarsi four-segmented, antennae usually longer than body—Family Tittigoniidae
138b Tarsi three-segmented, 139
(Metcalf, 1954, p. 40)

It will be noticed that this parallel form makes strict use of a couplet form. Each type of Key has numerous variations in details. In fact as far back as 1922 Williamson complained that the "number of forms used is now limited apparently only by the number of authors publishing such keys . . ." (Williamson, 1922, p. 703).

Each of the major types of Keys has its particular attributes (Metcalf, 1954; Voss, 1952). The indented form is less economical of space but it is easier to read and to perceive how the groups are arranged. The parallel form, which is economical of space, makes more direct use of the couplet form. Some taxonomists believe this to be necessary for a good Key (Metcalf, 1954). The decision as to which form the taxonomist uses is probably based on these factors as well as the kind of Keys with which the author has become most acquainted.

History of Keys

The history of Keys in biology has been described by Voss (1952) quite adequately. Except where so stated, most of this section was derived from his work. Keys appeared quite early in the history of biology. Many of the early attempts to classify biological organisms tended to dichotomize groups of organisms and so took on the basic form of a Key. Although the first recorded attempt to classify organisms was made by the ancient Greeks (e.g., Aristotle and Theophrastus), it was not until the middle of the seventeenth century that systematic work in this area was attempted to any great extent. Several men almost simultaneously created hierarchical systems of classifications using characteristics of the organisms. However, Nehemiah Grew was the first person to realize that such a hierarchical system could be used to locate a specific organism. He clearly describes the idea of a Key in the second half of his book *Anatomy of Plants,* published in 1682. This part of his book was read before the Royal Society on November 9, 1679. The appendix is headed "Being a method proposed for the ready finding by the leaf and flower, to what sort any plant belongeth." In the appendix he clearly distinguishes between a taxonomic system and a method used to locate plants.

An identification Key knowingly based on artificial groupings was first developed by Lamarck in his *Flore Francaise,* published in 1778. In the 3rd edition which was co-authored by A. P. de Candolle it is stated that the Key was a method that subdivides plants into artificial categories according to "contradictory" characteristics so as to lead the student to the name of the plant (Voss, 1952). This form of a Key, which involves the gradual subdividing of the total group by dichotomizing on the basis of certain characteristics, is the form Keys have taken in biology up to the present time. There have been few major changes in the keying method since then; one of them was the introduction of the indented method.

The first American to produce a Key was Alphonso Wood in 1845. Probably the best known American manual of botany using a Key was that of Asa Gray. He first used the word "Key" in referring to this method for locating a species in his book *A Manual of the Botany of the Northern United States,* published in 1848 (Voss, 1952).

Today Keys are used in all branches of biology to identify species. Although they generally vary in details almost all of them utilize either the parallel or indented form described above (Voss, 1952).

Recent Developments

In the last few decades the primary developments in taxonomy appear not to have involved Keys directly (Gilmore, 1951). However, some of these developments are relevant to the creation of a brain damage Key and so they will be discussed briefly.

From the time of Darwin most taxonomic theories conceived of the various classes as representing the products of evolution. Closely related taxonomic groups were considered to be phylogenetically related. In the process of evolution the similar taxonomic groups were thought to have diverged from a common ancestor more recently than groups that were taxonomically less alike. In essence the taxonomic groupings were thought to represent the top of the familiar evolutionary tree (Gilmore, 1951). The attempt, of course, was to make the taxonomic categories representative of genealogical derivation.

Although criticism dates as far back as Adamson's classification of mollusca in 1763 (Sneath, 1962), the criticism of this theory became widespread only recently. The basic criticism is that biologists often cannot determine what the genealogical relationship of an organism is, and so another theory of classification must be used. This criticism is particularly potent in regard to microorganisms, especially viruses (Sneath, 1962). Gilmore (1940, 1951) argues that organisms should be grouped according to "natural" classes, by which he means that the members of the class should have a great deal of overall affinity or similarity in regard to all their phenotypical characteristics. Sneath (1962) calls this kind of grouping "phenetic." This natural classification system may be related to the phylogenetic development of animals as Sokal and Sneath (1963) demonstrated, but generally such a relationship is an assumption since the only direct evidence of genealogical relationships comes from paleontology and consequently such evidence is relatively rare (Sokal & Sneath, 1963).

From the point of view of classifying brain damage, the natural or phenetic theory permits application of the methods of biological taxonomy whereas the genealogical concept would have been incompatible with such an application since brain damage does not evolve.

A third form of classification is the artificial grouping, in which the categorizing is based on a single feature such as size. The method used to classify any object is dependent on the purpose for the classification. Thus for some purposes an artificial classification such as "organisms that live above timberline" is very useful. The advantage of the natural classification, however, is that it serves the most purposes and thus has the greatest utility (Gilmore, 1951). Another way of stating this is that natural classifications contain much more information than artificial ones since they are based on many characteristics rather than one (Sokal & Sneath, 1963).

Accompanying this change in theory has been the development of a new approach to the mechanics of taxonomy itself. This development is the introduction of what Sneath (1962) calls polythetic classes. Beckner (1959) first described this concept, though he called it "polytypic." Sneath (1962) changed the name because he claimed the word "polytypic" already referred to a different kind of concept. The usual and traditional systems of taxonomy were monothetic. Monothetic groups are explained by Sokal and Sneath as follows: "The ruling idea of monothetic groups is that they are formed by rigid and successive logical divisions so that the possession of a unique set of features is both sufficient and necessary for membership in the group thus defined. They are called monothetic because the defining set of features is unique" (Sokal & Sneath, 1963, p. 13). That is, in a monothetic system a single characteristic or set of characteristics defines a group. These characteristics are both necessary and sufficient to constitute the group. Thus all members of the group must have all of these characteristics in the set to be classified in that group.

"A polythetic arrangement, on the other hand, places together organisms that have the greatest number of shared features, and no single feature is either essential to group membership or is sufficient to make an organism a member of the group" (Sokal & Sneath, 1963, p. 14). In a polythetic grouping it is simply the holding of a large number of characteristics in common that defines the group. No single characteristic or limited set of characteristics is essential for the definition of the group. Thus two groups might easily have many characteristics in common, but each member of a group would have more of the particular characteristics of its group than would members of any alternate group. Sneath believes that when the groups are established there will be discontinuatives so that one group will not merge into another one as occurs in a continuum (Sneath, 1962).

More precisely Beckner (1959, p. 22) conceives of a polythetic ("polytypic") class as a group in which

(a) each member "possesses a large (but unspecified) number of properties" in the group;
(b) each property "is possessed by large numbers of these individuals";
(c) no property is necessarily possessed by every member of the group.

The advantage of a polythetic group is that aberrant individuals are still included. Sokal and Sneath have explained the details of this procedure in their book *Principles of Numerical Taxonomy* (1963). The advantage of the monothetic system is that it is easier to construct without the aid of computers and that it readily lends itself to the construction of keys.

Keys, however, can be made to correspond to the polythetic classification system which is of special importance in the construction of a Key for brain damage. For instance, in using a battery of tests to determine which side of the brain is damaged probably no one test could accurately lateralize more than, say, 65% of the cases. Adding another test may increase this percentage to 75% and a whole battery of 10 tests could increase it to 85 or 90%. Any two of the 10 tests might be sufficient to indicate lateralized damage. No particular set of tests is necessary for the assessment, and so the method is polythetic. This is, in fact, the nature of the Halstead index. The Keys presented in this report also utilized this method to a great extent. Sneath (1962) discussed this problem in some detail. Keys need to utilize as few features as possible for convenience but they could be constructed to use several features, any one of which would be sufficient to enable one to move to the next step in the Key.

Sneath (1962) states that the frequency of occurrence for any characteristic could be computed as the percentage of individuals in a group in which a certain characteristic occurs. If it occurs in one-half of the cases, the percentage would be 50%. A measure could be computed that consists of the difference between the percentage of occurrence of a characteristic in two groups. Thus, if it occurred 50% in one group and 4% in another group, the obtained frequency would be 46%. The most useful characteristics for building a Key would be ones that occurred 0% in one group and 100% in another, for example, with a frequency of 1.0. Sneath feels that if several features had a frequency of .90 then together they would have sufficient reliability to construct a Key. Thus it appears possible to construct a polythetic Key as well as a monothetic one.

PSYCHOLOGICAL APPROACHES TO A KEY

In recent years the recognition that conventional statistics could not adequately handle patterns of data or profiles like the one used in MMPI analyses has led to the creation of nonstatistical objective approaches. Two of the earlier methods were the sign approach, such as Wechsler's signs of brain damage (Wechsler, 1944, p. 150) and the Halstead impairment index (Halstead, 1947). More recently several psychological "keying" systems which utilize an ordered set of rules for categorizing various kinds of psychological materials have been developed. Almost any categorizing system designed to be used with a computer has at least some elements of a Key. There are also several other attempts to construct nonstatistical methods of categorizing in the literature which might be considered to be methods of keying, at least in part.

Computer Programs

Several computer programs have been discussed in the literature. Piotrowski (1964) attempted to construct a method for a computer interpretation of the Rorschach. Most programs, however, have been applied to the MMPI which has a form that invites such an application. An MMPI program has been described by Finney (1966). This is essentially an uncomplicated method in which the scores on various scales are directly linked to verbal statements. There is evidently some use of two scales jointly but no pattern reading is attempted.

Kleinmuntz (1963) has described a rather complicated process that can be utilized to derive a computer program from an expert's vocalized reasoning concerning MMPI profiles. Unfortunately the rules used in his system were not published so it is difficult to determine whether they constitute a fully developed Key that might be compared to the Meehl-Dahlstrom rules (Meehl & Dahlstrom, 1960a, 1960b) or the Keys used in this study.

Nonlinear Systems

Meehl (1959) classified several objective systems for categorizing psychotic patients as nonlinear systems to distinguish this type of analysis from the more usual statistical methods. None of these systems made use of traditional statistical principles, though only the Meehl-Dahlstrom rules approached the form of a developed Key.

Much of this work appears to have derived from the Hathaway coding system (Hathaway, 1947) and this was one of the systems that Meehl discussed. Sullivan and Welsh (1952) suggested another system based on the comparative heights of the MMPI scales taken in pairs. If this comparative difference reached a certain cutting point it was considered a sign of a particular psychological process. The signs could be derived statistically and a cutting point, consisting of a designated number of signs, could be set as a kind of index to categorize a case. Taulbee and Sissons (1957) applied this system to separate psychotic from neurotic patients, with some success. At about that same time Lykken (1956) used mathematical concepts to construct a system of classifying coded MMPI profiles into one of several hundred separate cells. A certain number of these cells could be considered as containing psychotic codes and in time an index was formed for diagnosing psychosis. Essentially a categorizing system was established.

All of these, along with the statistical method, linear discriminant function, were compared both to the Meehl-Dahlstrom rules (1960a) and to clinical judgment in a study by Meehl (1959). In this study the accuracy of the clinical judgment varied from person to person. The Meehl-Dahlstrom rules appeared to be the most accurate of the systems compared, while the best clinical judgment only approached that of the Meehl-Dahlstrom rules in predictive accuracy. Several other studies have also testified to the accuracy of the Meehl-Dahlstrom rules (Meehl & Dahlstrom, 1960a; Heinrichs, 1964, 1966).

Of all the nonstatistical objective methods so far published the Meehl-Dahlstrom rules (Meehl & Dahlstrom, 1960a, 1960b) for Discriminating Psychotic from Neurotic MMPI Profiles appear to be the most sophisticated procedure. Essentially it takes the form of a loosely connected key and could easily be called "a key for psychoticism" (Meehl & Dahlstrom, 1960b). Probably its Key form is the aspect that enabled it to discriminate psychotics from neurotics better than other objective or clinical methods.

Suggested Systems

At least two objective nonlinear systems which were applied to brain damage have been suggested in the literature. One of these is the method of "successive sieves" suggested by Wechsler (1958). In this system a series of cutting points would be applied to a group of test results rather than a single cutting point. This method forms part of the essential nature of a Key in which criteria are applied serially rather than combined to form a single cutting point. This method was put to a test by Ladd (1964) who was able to correctly separate 72% of brain damaged from neurotic subjects on the basis of WAIS performance alone.

The final system is that described by Haynes and Sells (1963) which they attribute to W. C. Becker. Becker thought that diagnosis of brain damage should be a sequential decision-making process that was both multidimensional and hierarchically ordered. The initial decision would be whether brain damage exists; then the location and type of brain damage would be determined by successive decisions. This procedure is in the exact form of a Key and as such he was suggesting the manner in which a Key for brain damage might be constructed. Up to this point this suggested system had not been incorporated into a functioning method or Key.

There are other actuarial attempts to assess certain psychological material such as Marks and Seeman's (1963) thorough analysis of abnormal MMPI profiles. This material, however, does not appear to have been placed in the form of a published key.

CHAPTER 3

Rationale

Most of the concepts incorporated into the Keys to be described were based on expressed "inferential" material or on research hypotheses derived from several neuropsychologists. They were not based primarily on published research. Indirectly, however, all of the concepts were based on the research findings of Halstead, Reitan and other neuropsychologists, as well as on relevant neurological concepts such as cerebral dominance and contralateral control of sensory and motor functions.

The term neuropsychology should be defined. Neuropsychology, broadly defined, is the study of brain-behavior relationships (Pribram, 1962); that is, it is the study of the functioning of the brain. Usually human brain functioning is implied, but any study on subhuman organisms that might lead to a better understanding of human brain functioning is also included. As such, this field overlaps with physiological psychology, neurology, and the area of clinical psychology that deals with brain damage. More narrowly defined, neuropsychology is concerned with the application of psychological tests and procedures to the study of brain functioning. Most of the studies utilized in this research fall within the narrower definition, and the procedures of Halstead and Reitan constitute a major effort in this area.

DOMINANCE

Crucial to the understanding of human brain functioning is the concept of dominance. Until relatively recently the hemisphere of the brain which controlled the dominant hand was called the dominant hemisphere. It was also thought that this hemisphere contained the speech area of the brain. Thus, in right-handed people, the left or contralateral side of the brain was thought to be dominant, and the reverse was true for left-handed people. Penfield (Penfield & Roberts, 1959) challenged this concept on the basis of direct electrical stimulation of the brain during surgery designed to relieve epileptic seizures. He concluded that handedness had almost no relationship to the hemisphere in which speech was located; it was located in the left hemisphere in most cases regardless of handedness.

A more recent research review by Piercy (1964) has indicated that the problem of dominance is rather involved. While speech is controlled by the left side of the brain in almost all right-handed people, left-handedness is complicated. Often more precise examination reveals that "left-handed people" actually have a mixed handedness or incomplete dominance. Although most left-handed people apparently have the speech center on the left side of the brain, a significant proportion have a bilateral representation that accompanies their incomplete dominance. Teuber (1962) thinks that the term dominance is no longer meaningful when applied to the cerebral hemispheres and should be abandoned.

In any case, definite lateralization of the speech center can only be determined at present by surgical procedures which are seldom applied. The Keys in this study have assumed that regardless of handedness the left hemisphere controls speech. The exceptions to this were probably quite minor and in any case would have affected only a few of the tests in the battery.

LOCALIZATION CONTROVERSY

One of the assumptions of these Keys is that to a certain extent functions are localized in the brain. This assumption runs contrary to certain theories concerning brain functioning. This localization controversy is as old as the field of neurology itself (Boring, 1950). In relatively recent years the school of thought that did not accept strict cerebral localization was led by K. Goldstein (Goldstein, 1939, 1948; Goldstein & Scheerer, 1941). He was opposed by many neurologists. The various issues in this controversy go beyond the scope of this volume. A good review of this controversy, however, is given by Meyer (1961).

In regard to this controversy some of Reitan's work is quite important. He has attacked the position of Goldstein and Scheerer (1941) in order to establish a basis for his work, since his testing methods assume both localization of brain functioning and a quantitative difference between normal and brain damaged people (Reitan, 1956, 1958a, 1959d, 1966). Much of Reitan's later work (Reitan, 1966) has been devoted to the study of localized brain damage, especially lateralization. In any case, the concept of moderate localization of function in the brain has been generally accepted by neurology today. The last serious defense of cerebral equipotentiality may be found in Smith's (1962a) analysis of several difficulties encountered in research in brain damage, and this was not a strong endorsement. The position Smith took was not that brain tissue was totally equipotential.

He conceded that localization of function exists for the various sensory and motor modalities, but that many concepts of localization are oversimplified, mechanistic and not consistent with current research findings.

LATERALIZING STUDIES

Ever since Broca's work on the speech center (Boring, 1950) certain general mental functions have been considered to be lateralized in the human brain. The area that controlled speech was thought to be located in the dominant hemisphere or more recently in the left hemisphere, regardless of hand preference. The problems have been primarily (a) to determine exactly where in the left hemisphere speech was located, and (b) what was located in the right hemisphere. There are several good reviews of this question (Bauer & Wepman, 1955, Meyer, 1961, Piercy, 1964) so that here only recent findings and those pertinent to this study will be examined.

Sensory and Motor Functions

Before dealing with the lateralization of higher functions the known facts relating to basic sensory and motor functions may be mentioned since many of the individual tests used in the battery rely on this knowledge. The items that are mentioned here can be found in much greater detail in any textbook on neurology such as that by Elliott (1963).

Motor functioning in humans is controlled by many areas of the brain. From the point of view of the Key, however, the motor strip rostral to the central sulcus is most important. The functioning of this area is reflected directly in the Finger Tapping Test. In spite of its simplicity this is one of the most sensitive tests for brain damage, especially lateralized damage, in the entire battery (Reitan, 1964a).

The functioning of the sensory areas of the brain are examined by the group of tests which make up the perceptual disorders examination. Gross dysfunctions are reflected in anesthesias and hypesthesias while the more subtle deficits are reflected in suppression phenomena (i.e., impairment of perception on double simultaneous stimulation when perception of single stimuli is intact). Sensory areas are located in several postcentral parts of the cortex which cover the anterior parietal and temporal lobes and the occipital pole.

The major principle related to both motor and sensory functioning is that of contralateral representation (i.e., the motor and sensory representation in the brain is opposite its location in the body). The left hemisphere controls the right hand and so forth. This does not hold strictly for all senses but these complications are also built into the Key. Thus, in regard to vision, contralaterality holds for visual fields rather than for eyes and in regard to hearing the auditory representation appears to be bilateral.

These lateralizing sensory deficits were investigated in several studies by Reitan (1958b), Wheeler & Reitan (1962). Although many patients who had lateralized brain damage failed to demonstrate deficits on the various sensory-perceptual tests that Reitan added to the battery, when these effects did occur they were almost always accurate indications of lateralized damage.

Speech

Recent work on the speech area of the brain has led to a more exact determination of its location and some of this work was incorporated into the Localization Key. Probably the most thorough attempt to localize parts of the brain controlling speech has been reported by Penfield and Roberts (1959). They locate three areas all on the left side of the brain: (a) Broca's area, (b) Wernicke's area (which is at the end of the lateral fissure and extends down into the temporal lobe) and (c) a supplementary area on the superior margin of the left hemisphere. These areas are extensive enough so that almost any fairly large degree of brain pathology on the left side of the brain should affect one of them. An excellent review of the various aphasias is given by Piercy (1964).

Reitan has made use of this knowledge to develop an aphasia test that is sensitive to left hemisphere damage. This test was incorporated into the Key. It is a modification of the Halstead and Wepman (1949) aphasia screening test. Using brain damaged patients with right and left homonymous visual field defects, brain damaged patients without visual field defects and normal controls, Doehring and Reitan (1961) found that the verbal parts of the examination lateralized to the left since they were correlated with a right visual field defect. The part of the test having to do with the drawing of geometric forms (i.e., the nonverbal spatial relations test) lateralized to the right. Wheeler and Reitan (1962) confirmed these results and developed a set of rules, which are essentially sign cutting points, to predict right and left cerebral damage. Also, a brief examination which used parts of the Aphasia Test to lateralize brain damage was constructed by Heimburger and Reitan (1961).

Recent studies have attempted to determine whether speech has any bilateral representation. One of the primary sources of information came from patients who have whole cerebral hemispheres removed due to tumors or infantile hemiplegia. Such a hemispherectomy can prolong the life of a person with a fast growing tumor or relieve infantile hemiplegia due to the agenesis of one cerebral hemisphere. There are several older reviews of hemispherectomies (Gardner, Karnosh, McClure & Gardner, 1955); however, the use of psychological tests in this area is relatively new

(Bruell & Albee, 1962) and the most thorough report of psychological testing published is quite recent (Smith & Burklund, 1966). Although the entire left hemisphere was removed, the right-handed patient retained comprehension of speech even though initially he could not talk. Gradually speech returned and he became able to do simple arithmetic. Thus location of speech appears to be more a matter of degree of lateralization than of absolute lateralization.

These results were reinforced from another source in the last few years. The split brain preparation which was developed by Sperry (1961) has led to a better understanding of brain functioning. This procedure has been applied when such a sectioning of the cerebral commissure was found to be beneficial to patients with intractable epilepsy. Earlier studies (Van Wagener & Harren, 1940) had led to the conclusion that cutting this cerebral commissure had no behavioral effects. Apparently this was an example of the concept that effects are not found unless there are tests for them. In the studies by Sperry and his co-workers elaborate psychological techniques were utilized and effects were found. Gazzaniga and Sperry (1967) demonstrated that speaking in man is controlled by the left hemisphere but apparently both hemispheres can comprehend speech, at least to a certain extent. This was roughly the same conclusion as that of Smith and Burklund's (1966) study of a hemispherectomy.

Right Hemisphere Functions

For many years the function of the nondominant hemisphere was not known except for the contralateral control of the sensory and motor systems. In 1939 Hebb published a study that indicated the kind of special function found in the right hemisphere. Since then a great many studies have confirmed the nonverbal type of function located there. The items on the Halstead-Wepman aphasia examination that indicate right-sided damage are simple drawings. The most sensitive of these is a Greek cross. Kløve and Reitan (1958) demonstrated that brain damaged patients who had trouble drawing the Greek cross and thus supposedly had right cerebral damage also did more poorly on the performance items of the Wechsler-Bellevue intelligence examination than on the verbal items. This indicated that the performance items, and especially the Block Design, were related to right hemisphere functioning.

More recent work has attempted to determine the nature of this lateralized function more precisely. A study on humans with the cerebral commissures split for therapeutic purposes (Gazzaniga, Bogen & Sperry, 1965) demonstrated that three-dimensional spatial relations concepts are mediated by the right hemisphere. Even though the subject had more control over the execution of drawing with his right hand he could only copy a three-dimensional cube with his left such that the perspective was retained. Semmes, Weinstein, Ghent and Teuber (1963) were able to show that there are at least two kinds of spatial orientation found in man, only one of which, extrapersonal, is located in the right posterior hemisphere. Body localization was found to be located in the left posterior cortex. Many other studies (Teuber, 1962, 1966; Milner, 1962; Warrington & James, 1967) are gradually separating out the kinds of functions located in the right hemisphere. However, this material was not utilized in the Keys that are part of this study.

Intelligence Studies

A large number of studies have originated in Reitan's laboratory which deal with lateralization effects on the Wechsler-Bellevue. Some earlier research had indicated that the Wechsler-Bellevue subscales were not differentially affected by brain damage (Cohen, 1955). Hewson's ratios (Hewson, 1949), which numerically compare various scales against one another, were found to be fairly effective by several investigators (Smith, 1962b; Wolff, 1960) in indicating the presence of brain damage, thus demonstrating that subtest patterns were affected by it. These ratios make a great deal of use of the Digit Symbol Test which became part of the battery used in these studies.

In 1959 Reitan (1959a) demonstrated that performance on the Wechsler-Bellevue Test was affected by brain damage, though not as much as the Halstead index. Wechsler's "hold" (Vocabulary, Information, Object Assembly, Picture Completion) and "don't hold" (Digit Span, Similarities, Digit Symbol and Block Design) tests were not significantly affected. Then a series of studies demonstrated that right hemisphere damage affected the performance part of the Wechsler-Bellevue Test and left hemisphere lesions depressed the verbal scales (Reitan, 1955a; Doehring & Reitan, 1962; Reitan, 1964a; Reed & Reitan, 1963). The first study showing these effects had been done by Andersen in 1950. This difference appeared whether the subjects were selected on the basis of aphasia (Kløve & Reitan, 1958; Reitan, 1960), homonymous visual field defects (Doehring, Reitan & Kløve, 1961), electroencephalograph patterns (Kløve, 1959a), or sensory suppression (Kløve, 1959b). Finally a factor analysis of the Wechsler-Bellevue subtests gave a right-performance and a left-verbal factor as well as factors for normals and hysterics (Matthews, Guertin & Reitan, 1962).

In the Key used in the present study this difference was utilized in setting up a ratio between three of the verbal tests: Digit Span, Similarities, and Vocabulary and two performance tests; Block Design and Object Assembly. These tests were selected since inspection of research results on the Wechsler Test demonstrated them to be the most sensitive tests to lateralization (Kløve & Reitan, 1958). There may be some difference, however, between the WAIS results used in this study and the Wechsler-Bellevue results from which this ratio was originally taken (Fitzhugh & Fitzhugh, 1964a). Further investigation should be utilized to determine if such a difference does exist and to change the ratio in accordance with it.

PROCESS STUDIES

Some studies contradicted the above results by finding no difference between verbal and performance subtests in spite of lateralized cerebral damage (Kløve & Fitzhugh, 1962). This contradiction, however, was explained when it was found that although there was a verbal-performance discrepancy in acute brain damage cases this difference does not occur in old static cases of brain damage (Fitzhugh, Fitzhugh & Reitan, 1961, 1962a, 1962b). This lack of difference for static brain damage was true for the WAIS as well as the Wechsler-Bellevue Test (Fitzhugh & Fitzhugh, 1964a, 1964b). Rennick, G. Goldstein and others have promulgated the hypothesis that acute brain damage would tend to be severe and highly lateralized, whereas static brain damage would be moderate and diffuse. This concept was incorporated into the Process Key.

The Key pattern that was utilized for congenital brain damage was derived from acquaintance with the neuropsychological "inferential" rules for determining this form of brain damage. These were evidently part of general neurological knowledge. Some of this knowledge had been formed into hypotheses by G. Goldstein which have been investigated in his laboratory.

CHAPTER 4

The Neuropsychological Keys

Two major Keys for categorizing brain damage were developed for this study. The Localization Key was designed for determining the existence and lateralization of brain damage. This Key separates cases into four categories: (a) no brain damage, (b) diffuse brain damage, (c) right hemisphere damage, (d) left hemisphere damage. An additional section of this first Key was designed to indicate the *degree* of lateralization. It is in fact a separate, though minor, Key.

The Process Key was designed to determine the type of brain damage that the subject had. Again four categories were used: (a) no brain damage, (b) acute brain damage, (c) static brain damage, and (d) congenital brain damage. In general, rapidly progressive brain lesions would be included in the acute category, and slowly progressive lesions would be included under the static category. The Process Key presupposes both the Localization Key as well as the Degree of Lateralization Key.

In this chapter the list of tests used is presented, as well as information about the construction of the Keys. This material is followed by a presentation of the Keys themselves and some examples of how they are applied to specific cases.

LIST OF TESTS

The following is a complete list of tests which are part of the neuropsychological test battery that G. Goldstein utilizes and which were a part of this study:

1. Average Impairment rating.
*2. Halstead Category test.
3. Halstead Tactual Performance test (TPT) (Speed) dominant hand.
4. Halstead Tactual Performance test (Speed) nondominant hand.
5. Halstead Tactual Performance test (Speed) both hands.

* Tests used to obtain the average impairment rating.

*6. Halstead Tactual Performance test (Speed) total.
*7. Halstead Tactual Performance test (Memory).
*8. Halstead Tactual Performance test (Location).
*9. Seashore Rhythm test.
*10. Halstead Speech Perception test.
*11. Halstead Finger Tapping—dominant hand.
12. Halstead Finger Tapping—nondominant hand.
13. Trail Making A
*14. Trail Making B
*15. Digit Symbol test from WAIS (rating).
*16. Aphasia examination (rating).
*17. Spatial Relations examination (rating).
*18. Perceptual Disorders examination (rating).
19. Finger Agnosia—right hand.
20. Finger Agnosia—left hand.
21. Finger Tip Writing—right hand.
22. Finger Tip Writing—left hand.
23. Tactual Hypesthesia—right hand.
24. Tactual Hypesthesia—left hand.
25. Suppression, visual—right field.
26. Suppression, visual—left field.
27. Suppression, auditory—right ear.
28. Suppression, auditory—left ear.
29. Suppression, Tactual—right hand and face.
30. Suppression, Tactual—left hand and face.
31. Homonymous Hemianopia—right field.
32. Homonymous Hemianopia—left field.
33. WAIS—Full Scale IQ.
34. WAIS—Verbal IQ.
35. WAIS—Performance IQ.
36. Vocabulary subtest.
37. Digit Span subtest.
38. Similarities subtest.
39. Block Design subtest.
40. Object Assembly subtest.
41. Lateral Dominance examination.

CONSTRUCTION OF THE KEYS

The central problem in constructing the Keys was to translate the inferential concepts or rules that neuropsychologists use "intuitively" into objective statements. Originally, the form of the biological key appeared to be similar to the kind of inferential process that psychologists use when they employ clinical intuition in arriving at a conclusion. When the steps included in the inferential process are separated and written down, as they rarely are, the resemblance between the clinical inferential process and the logical system of a Key becomes apparent. In order to demonstrate this similarity, an example of the reasoning of a neuropsychologist will be used. The following passage is an abridged version of a case analysis presented by Reitan (1966).

The extremely poor performance of W. C. on Halstead's tests and the Trail Making Test, together with the strong lateralizing indications, strongly suggested a type of lesion that has grossly impairing effects. The likely possibilities, in these terms, were either a cerebral neoplasm or a vascular accident. . . . A particular point of information from the test results, however, strongly indicated a neoplasm. This information came particularly from a comparison of the severity of impairment of higher-level functions associated with damage of the right hemisphere and the severity of impairment of motor functions. Higher-level functions, as described above, were severely impaired in this patient. He also demonstrated some impairment of motor functions of the left upper extremity, although this impairment was less pronounced. This combination of factors lean our differential inference very much in the direction of a neoplastic lesion. While the observation stands in need of experimental study, our past experiences indicate that severe impairment of higher-level functions relating to lateralized cerebral damage is much more frequently accompanied by profound motor deficits in the case of cerebral vascular lesions than with cerebral tumors. . . .

After we reached this point in the interpretation of the results, a final consideration was necessary regarding whether the neoplasm was primary or metastatic. As far as we could judge from present insights based upon past experiences, our only prospect for achieving this differentiation related to the need for postulating more than one lesion to explain the test results. The likelihood of more than one lesion is far less for primary gliomas than for metastatic neoplasms. Our prospects for inferring two structurally separate lesions in one hemisphere are slim, but we not infrequently obtain evidence suggesting the presence of a structural lesion in each cerebral hemisphere. . . . However, patient W. C. did demonstrate clear right-left confusion, mild difficulties in finger localization on the right hand and a pronounced tendency to misinterpret and confuse signs of specific arithmetical operations such as + and −. These deficits are much more frequently an indication of left than right cerebral damage (Wheeler and Reitan, 1962). (The main lesion had been located on the right.)

On this basis we suspected that a lesion of the left cerebral hemisphere was present (which was much less significant than the lesion on the right side) and correspondingly leaned our interpretation slightly in favor of metastatic cerebral neoplasm. Although clinical neurological findings did not confirm our inference of a possible left cerebral lesion, histological examination revealed that the lesion was an epidermoid carcinoma, metastatic from the lung. (Reitan, 1966, pp. 200–201.)

This reasoning, when placed in the form of a Key, would be roughly as follows: (The items that were not used in the reasoning are not filled in.)

I. Generalized impairment
  A. – – – –
  B. – – – –
II. Localized impairment
  A. Higher level functions mild to moderately impaired (e.g., Categories and Trail Making Tests).
    1. – – – –
    2. – – – –
  B. Higher level functions severely impaired (e.g., extremely poor performance on Categories and Trail Making).
    1. Motor impairment relative to higher level functions quite severe. CEREBRAL VASCULAR LESION
      a. – – – –
      b. – – – –
    2. Motor impairment relative to higher level functions mild or moderate. CEREBRAL NEOPLASM
      a. Evidence for multiple lesions (e.g., functions located in two or more areas affected). METASTATIC NEOPLASM
      b. Evidence for a single lesion. PRIMARY NEOPLASM—(glioma)

In this Key it will be observed that at each level possibilities are reduced until the position "II B 2 a" is arrived at, giving a diagnosis of cerebral metastatic neoplasm.

Sources for Parts of the Keys

The sources for material used to build the Keys were quite varied and are only mentioned briefly here. Since much of the inferential process used in neuropsychological diagnosis is not made explicit in the literature, a great deal of information was obtained through attendance at lectures and workshops offered by neuropsychologists, particularly Dr. Rennick at the Menninger Foundation. Rennick presented a number of "rules of thumb" used by himself and other neuropsychologists to determine existence, location and type of process in brain damage. Second, G. Goldstein's reports on cases examined at the Topeka Veterans Administration Hospital usually were found to contain part of the reasoning behind his diagnosis. These rationales for diagnostic conclusions concerning individual cases were generalized into working rules that were ultimately formulated into Key statements. There are also several studies reported in the literature which contain statistical information that contributed to construction of the Key. Some of these studies enabled the present authors to fix some of the criteria more exactly than might otherwise have been possible. These studies are discussed in Chapter 3 in the section in which the rationale for the Keys is presented.

The Process of Constructing the Keys

The actual construction of the Keys was a cyclical process. First a group of rules were brought together without set criteria and ordered in a rough manner. Fortunately, Reitan had previously constructed a set of hypotheses concerning diagnosis of various aspects of brain damage (Reitan, 1959c). Most of these hypotheses were based on experimental evidence, and many of them had to do with the question of lateralization. They were used to form the nucleus of the Localization Key. The first attempt at a key was applied to a group of cases in a preliminary pilot study. Results were encouraging, but changes had to be made in both the order of rules and in the rules themselves. Cutting points were then set and the Keys applied to another series of cases. The results were quite similar to those to be reported for the present study. Additional minor changes were made and the Keys were applied to the cases reported here. Both the Localization and Process Keys were developed by the same procedure. However, the Process Key is not so fully developed as the Localization Key since neurological confirmation of process is generally more difficult to diagnose than is determination of localization.

Modifications of the Neuropsychological Battery for the Keys

In order to apply the key method to the Halstead Battery and related procedures, it was necessary to make modifications in both the traditional Key form and the scoring system used for the test battery. Two objectives were sought; transformation of the key method into an accurate and viable instrument for categorizing brain damage, and objectification of the procedure to the extent that no person more highly skilled than the technician who does the testing and scoring would be needed to arrive at the final diagnostic statement. The aim was to construct the Key operations such that a technician or clerk, without knowledge of neurology, neuropsychology or psychometrics, could begin with the test results and run the Key through to the final diagnostic classification. It was, in fact, an aim of this project to determine whether or not the Keys could be sufficiently objectified to make this feasible. It was also felt that the objectification of the scoring and inferential systems used might ultimately lead to computer interpretation of the neuropsychological battery. A computer program for the Keys is presented in the Appendix of this book. This program can be adapted to refinements and modifications of the Key.

From almost the beginning of the attempt to construct neuropsychological Keys, it was obvious that there could be no strict adherence to the form of the biological key. Evidently, the inferential process, while often quite analogous to the form of a biological key, sometimes deviates from this form. Another problem that had to be taken into account was the greater variability in consequences of brain damage than in types of organisms.

The effect of these two factors on the construction of the Neuropsychological Keys led to abandonment of the traditional couplet form. The final form of the Keys used in this study is quite complex since it had to be of the polythetic variety and because of the complexity of the inferential process used in neuropsychological diagnosis. It will be recalled that in the polythetic method, movement from one step of the Key to another is frequently based on many indicators, none of which are either necessary or sufficient. Only the required or stated combination is necessary or sufficient; for example, in the case of lateralizing brain damage, a variety of indicators may be involved, such as paralysis of one side of the body, sensory defect and speech impairment. In fact, determination of left hemisphere brain damage by the Localization Key involves certain combinations of as many as thirteen different indicators. It is this polythetic characteristic that gives the Key a great deal of its predictive power.

The reasoning process used by neuropsychologists is not only fairly intricate but also varies in its characteristics from step to step. Thus it did not appear to be feasible to retain any consistent form of logic from step to step. The form of the resulting key was rather far from the elegance that mathematicians prefer, but future versions may reduce this awkwardness of style. A practical result of this complexity was that it became necessary to build instructions into the Key itself at almost every step. These instructions tell the reader how to proceed and give the logic of the next step.

Modifications in Scoring the Neuropsychological Battery

In the process of constructing the Neuropsychological Keys, it was found that certain changes in scoring of the battery had to be made. As indicated above, the initial scoring system for the battery was developed by Halstead, modified by Reitan and modified further by Rennick. The system devised by Rennick, particularly that part of it involving the Average Impairment Rating, was the one modified for the Key.

Only one change was made in regard to what tests were included in computation of the Average Impairment Rating. The change concerned the Finger Tapping Test. In Halstead's (1947) and Reitan's (1966) studies tapping speed of the dominant hand only was included in the Impairment Index. The difficulty with this procedure is that tapping speed reflects, for the most part, the state of the brain contralateral to the tapping hand. Although there is some ipsilateral control of the motor system, it plays a very minor role for the hands. Thus a person with right hemisphere brain damage could maintain normal tapping speed for his right hand, and if he happens to be right hand dominant, this normal score would be included in the Impairment Index rather than the abnormal score he obtains with his left hand. For this reason the tapping speed of the most impaired hand was used in computing the Average Impairment Rating, rather than the speed of the dominant hand.

Another modification of the scoring system involved extension of the available norms. Norms were not available for each trial of the Tactual Performance Test (time for dominant hand, nondominant hand and both hands) since total time was the only speed score included in the Impairment Index. Thus new norms were constructed for each hand separately. Norms were not available for finger tapping with the nondominant hand and so they were also constructed. These new norms were based primarily on the "rules of thumb" that Rennick and others used to judge relative impairment of right and left hands in performing a task. It was also found that the Trail Making Test norms had to be rescaled, since the available norms tended to overestimate severity of deficit relative to other tests in the battery. By using the scores from Reitan's normative study of the Trail Making Test (Reitan, 1958c) the scaled score of "one" was set at the first standard deviation of the normal group. The scores of the brain damaged group that fell outside of this range were divided into four equal groups and assigned severity of impairment ratings accordingly. (For these new scales see Appendix A.)

The third major modification of the scoring system of the neuropsychological battery involved quantification of the Aphasia, Spatial Relations and Perceptual Disorders Tests. Performance on these tests had been rated on an intuitive basis by the neuropsychologist, the rating indicating how much he felt deficits in these areas contributed to the probability of there being brain damage. Quantitative scoring systems were substituted for these impressionistic ratings in keeping with the authors' aim of making the key usable by a clerk, technician, or computer.

As mentioned above, the Aphasia Test consisted of a modification of the Halstead-Wepman Aphasia Test. In the past the neuropsychologist listed the aphasic symptoms demonstrated by the patient and based his rating on the number and severity of symptoms. In order to quantify the scoring of this test, one of the authors (Goldstein) assigned a numerical score to each item on the test that had to do with language functioning. The drawings of the square, cross, triangle and key were not included. A weighted scoring system was used, with errors on certain items receiving only one point, whereas errors on other items could receive as many as four points. This weighting system was used because not all aphasic errors are equally serious. For example, inability to find the name of a shown object is far more serious than inability to spell that name correctly. Weighting was made on the basis of Goldstein's judgments concerning the degree of seriousness of an error on each of the items. The total number of error scores from a sample of 75 cases were separated into categories according to Goldstein's subjectively made degree of impairment ratings and cutting points for each of the scaled scores were set by inspection. The ranges of raw scores that fit into each of the scaled score categories were set in this manner. (See Appendices A and B.)

An attempt was made to establish the reliability of the new Aphasia Test scoring system. Thirty cases were randomly selected and were scored independently by three individuals, two of whom were trained neuropsychological technicians. These people normally administer the battery, but had no experience in rating the aphasia examination. The third person was one of the authors (Russell) who had only minimal experience in aphasia testing. Kendall's co-efficient of concordance (Siegel, 1956) was computed in order to evaluate degree of agreement among the three scores. A W of .88, which is significant at the .001 level and is equivalent to an average Pearson r of .82 was obtained. The validity of this scoring system was determined by comparing the mean score of the three scorers with Goldstein's subjective ratings. A Pearson r of .79 was obtained. It may be pointed out that the term validity, as used here, simply refers to extent of agreement with subjective ratings made by a neuropsychologist with regard to degree of aphasia.

The problem of quantifying the spatial relations test was substantially more difficult than was the case for the aphasia test. The procedure in the past had been for the neuropsychologist to inspect the drawings of the square, Greek cross, triangle and door key that the patient made as part of the Aphasia Test, and to rate them according to extent of distortion of the various spatial configurations. As supplementary data to be used in borderline cases, the neuropsychologist could also use the Block Design subtest of the WAIS and the drawing of the Halstead Tactual Performance

Test. In this evaluation, the most crucial item was the Greek cross. The other drawings usually prove to be nondiscriminating in adults, and the Block Design subtest is far from being a pure measure of spatial relations ability. Thus these latter tests were used only to change the rating by no more than one point in borderline cases, but the major consideration was always degree of distortion in the drawing of the cross.

To objectify this rating procedure the scoring method used by Graham and Kendall on their Memory for Designs Test was adopted (Graham & Kendall, 1960). A series of drawings of crosses taken from actual cases were categorized into three groups by Goldstein according to severity of deficit demonstrated. Typical examples of these drawings were collected into a manual to serve as models for use by unskilled raters. (See Appendix C.) To score a protocol, the drawing is matched against the samples in the manual and given a score of 1 to 5. [The zero rating (excellent) was not used as it appeared to be meaningless in this situation.] Since each subject was required to draw the cross twice, scores ranging from 2 to 10 could be obtained. Next, the WAIS Block Design subtest score was considered. If it was the lowest WAIS subtest score, with the exceptions of Object Assembly and Digit Symbol, then two points were added to the score. If not, no additional points were added or subtracted. A table that converts this raw score to a six-point scaled score was constructed in order to obtain the rating formerly made intuitively by the neuropsychologist. Thus an objective method was arrived at in order to rate spatial relations ability. (See Appendices A and C.)

The reliability of this scoring procedure was evaluated using the same judges and subject population as was used for the Aphasia Test. The examples contained in the manual were not produced by patients used in this report. Kendall's coefficient of concordance was .97, which is significant at the .001 level, and the equivalent average Pearson r was .95. The validity of the measure was once more determined by comparing the average of the three scores for each subject with Goldstein's independently made "intuitive" ratings. Pearson r was .92, indicating that the results obtained through the use of the objective scoring system closely approximated the ratings made subjectively by the neuropsychologist.

For the Perceptual Disorders Tests the neuropsychologist made a subjective, global rating of the extent to which various sensory and perceptual deficits contributed to overall extent of impairment. He used tests of finger-tip writing perception, finger discrimination, suppression on double simultaneous tactile, auditory and visual stimulation and the visual field examination (Reitan, 1966). With the exception of visual fields these tests yield quantitative scores, and so quantification of the global perceptual disorders rating could be accomplished in a straight-forward manner. However, since suppression is usually interpreted as a more serious symptom than impaired finger tip number writing or finger discrimination, errors on the tests for suppression were given a weighting of 1.5. The total raw score could then be obtained simply by counting errors. The raw scores of 70 cases were separated into categories according to Goldstein's rating of severity of impairment, and cutting points for each scaled score were set by inspection. This operation resulted in an objective scaled score for the perceptual disorders tests. (See Appendices A and D.)

The reliability of this scoring method was not evaluated since, except for clerical errors, there can be no discrepancy among scorers. Validity was determined by comparing the subjective ratings with the scored ratings, using a new sample of 30 cases. A Pearson *r* of .79 was obtained, which was sufficient for the purposes of this study.

A quantitative measure was also developed for the visual field examination. Its purpose was that of assigning scores to various homonymous field defects, that is, loss of vision in corresponding halves or quadrants of the visual field. The method is a fairly simple one and makes use of standard visual field examination charts. It consists of counting the number of squares in the right half of the chart for both eyes (right visual field) in which vision is preserved, making the same count for the left half of the chart and comparing the two. The criterion point of half as many functioning squares in one field as the other was adapted liberally from information contained in a standard text on the neurological examination (McDowell & Wolff, 1960). No attempt was made to validate this test since it is simply a convenient method of identifying visual field defects and can readily be used by a technician with no training in neurology. This technique was added to the Key since, although rare, homonymous field defects are almost always pathognomonic of lateralized brain damage.

There were also some other minor changes made in constructing the Keys. One of these involved the construction of a WAIS scale to predict right versus left hemisphere brain damage. In many studies the verbal weighted score of the Wechsler-Bellevue or the verbal IQ of the WAIS has been found to be depressed in association with left hemisphere brain damage, while the corresponding performance IQ measures were more effected by right hemisphere damage (Andersen, 1950; Fitzhugh & Fitzhugh, 1964a; Fitzhugh, Fitzhugh & Reitan, 1962a; Kløve, 1959a; Reitan, 1955a). Closer examination of some of these results demonstrated that some subtests were more vulnerable to lateralized brain damage than others (Kløve & Reitan, 1958). Consequently a more sensitive index might be constructed by using only these most sensitive verbal and performance tests for purposes of predicting lateralization. The verbal tests selected were Vocabulary, Digit Span and Similarities, while Block Design and Object

Assembly were the performance tests chosen. Although not as reliable, the Object Assembly subtest correlates more highly with Block Design than any other test in the WAIS, and in a study of chronically brain damaged patients it was the only test that was related to lateralized defect to a significant degree (Fitzhugh & Fitzhugh, 1964b). The index constructed from these three verbal and two performance subtests was not specifically validated. However, it was included in the Key and appeared to contribute to its results.

Finally, a scoring system was devised for the lateral dominance examination. It consisted of a measure for mixed dominance (absence of clearly differentiated handedness or eyedness) and crossed dominance (right handed and left eyed or vice versa). The lateral dominance examination consists of seven measures for handedness (one of them being given a weight of 3) and 10 trials for determination of eyedness (Miles ABC Test). Some other indicators, including tests for footedness are also routinely given but were not included in the Key. The measure developed consists of a count of indicators and a comparison of the dominant hand with the opposite eye. (See Appendix E.) The cutting points were set by reference to "rules of thumb." Since simple counting is all that is required, the reliability study was not appropriate. Although no validity measure was attempted, the presence of crossed or mixed lateral dominance was a good indicator for determination of congenital brain damage by the Process Key. This finding suggests that this new lateral dominance measure is meaningful in terms of its ability to predict brain dysfunction.

Instructions for Use of Keys

A. The Localization Key

The raw scores obtained from the various tests and their rating point equivalents are entered in a "Neuropsychology Summary Sheet." (The conversion tables used to obtain rating points will be found in Appendix A.)

In general, the key follows the outline method. One proceeds from major Roman numeral I to A to 1, etc. In the case of the Localization Key, if brain damage is established as present, it is necessary to proceed through the entire Key. The only exit before completion of the key is at the end of heading I, in the event that no brain damage is present. If brain damage is found to be present, running the key simply involves accumulating points for the left and right hemispheres and comparing point counts at the end. It should be made clear that if points are assigned for a particular test under the two-point indicators they are also assigned for that test under the one-point indicators; for example, if two points are assigned for impaired tapping speed as a two-point indicator (II A 1 b and II B 1 b), another point is assigned for the one-point tapping indicator (II A 2 C and II B 2 C) for a total of three points.

There are several additional features to notice. Sometimes the raw scores are more sensitive to brain dysfunction than are the ratings. Therefore some of the statements are written by using raw scores (e.g., II A 2 d 1). The user of the Key is cautioned to be aware of this distinction when he is making his point count. Attention is also called to the invalidation rules for the perceptual disorders tests. Certain minimum scores are required for the indicators to be assigned points, and in the case of the suppression tests, substantial impairment of the appropriate primary sensory function invalidates these indicators. In counting number of suppressions, count the total number for each side; that is, for tactual suppression total the hand and face scores; for visual suppression total the upper, middle and lower visual field scores. Sometimes patients have extensive lack of use of one side of their body, so much so that they are unable to perform certain of the tests at all. In these cases we have used the convention of indicating this with an *X*. An *X* score, however, does not invalidate the test. If, for example, the patient cannot do the tapping test at all with his right hand, two points are assigned for indicator II A 1 b.

B. The Degree of Lateralization Key

It should be pointed out that this Key may only be applied to those cases in which lateralized brain damage has been established by the Localization Key. The presence of a two point indicator for the hemisphere in which the damage has been lateralized by the Localization Key always means strong lateralization. If a two-point indicator is not present, three more one point indicators must be present on one side than on the other.

C. The Process Key

The Process Key presupposes the Localization and Degree of Lateralization Keys, since results obtained from these latter Keys are used as some of the Process Key's criteria. It differs from the Localization Key in that there are several exit points, one for each category. Therefore it is not necessary to proceed through the entire Key in all cases. As soon as the criterion for a given category is met the running of the Key should be stopped. For example, if an Average Impairment Rating of three or more is found and there are strong lateralizing signs, the case is classified as acute. Other scores and indices used as criteria in the other categories are not relevant to the identification of acute brain damage and so need not be examined.

The identification of mixed and crossed lateral dominance is made through the use of a Lateral Dominance Scale. (See Appendices A and E.)

THE NEUROPSYCHOLOGICAL KEYS [1]

A. The Localization Key

I. Determine presence or absence of brain damage.
   A. Criterion: Average Impairment Rating is less than 1.55
      NO BRAIN DAMAGE—STOP

II. If brain damage is present (Average Impairment Rating greater than or equal to 1.55) determine lateralization.
   A. Criterion for left hemisphere brain damage: The sum of all points lateralizing to the left hemisphere is at least twice as large as the sum of all points lateralizing to the right hemisphere. Indicators for left hemisphere brain damage:
      1. Two-point indicators
         a. The score for the Aphasia Test must be at least three rating points worse than the score for the Spatial Relations Test.
         b. Right-handed people must average more than five fewer taps with their right hand than with their left. Left-handed people must average more than 20 fewer taps with their right hand than with their left.
      2. One-point indicators
         a. The Aphasia Test score must be one rating point poorer than the Spatial Relations Test score.
         b. TPT-Right Hand time score must be worse than TPT-Left Hand time score by at least two rating points.
         c. For right-handed people tapping speed with the right hand must be slower than tapping speed with the left hand. For left-handed people tapping speed with the right hand must average more than 10 taps slower than with the left.
         d. There must be more impairment of sensory function on the right side of the body than on the left. This indicator is said to be present if any *one* of the following are present:
            (1) At least 2.5 times as many errors are made on the Finger Agnosia Test with the right hand as with the left. (Invalid if there are less than four errors with the right hand.)
            (2) At least 2.5 times as many errors are made on the Finger-Tip Number Writing Test with the right hand as with the left. (Invalid if there are less than six errors with the right hand.)
            (3) The rating for hypesthesia of the right side must be at least 2.5 times that obtained for the left side. (Invalid if the rating for the right hand is less than three.)
         e. Suppression on double simultaneous stimulation must be more severe on the right side than on the left. This indicator is said to be present if any *one* of the following is true:

[1] A formal version of these keys may be found in Appendix J.

(1) At least 2.5 times as many suppressions of the right ear are made than of the left ear on double simultaneous auditory stimulation. (Invalid if there are less than three suppressions of the right ear.)

(2) At least 2.5 times as many suppressions of tactual stimulation on the right side are made than on the left side on double simultaneous tactual stimulation. (Invalid if there are less than four suppressions on the right side.)

(3) At least 2.5 times as many suppressions of the right visual field than of the left visual field are found on double simultaneous visual stimulation. (Invalid if less than four suppressions of the right visual field.)

NOTE: Tests of suppression are invalid if the primary sensory functions are not relatively intact. Thus, if there is a hearing loss rated three or four in either ear, the auditory suppression test is invalidated; if there is a hypesthesia rated three or four for either hand, the tactual suppression test is invalidated; if there is loss of vision in the right or left visual field, the visual suppression test is invalidated. Loss of vision is evaluated by perimetric examination.

f. A right homonymous hemianopia is found. This indicator is said to be present if, on perimetric examination, the right visual field has half the number or less of functioning squares than the left visual field. Squares are counted on standard perimetric examination charts. (Invalid if the total number of functioning squares in both eyes is equal to or less than 96.)

g. On the WAIS there must be more impairment on the verbal tests than on the performance tests. This indicator is present if a prorated verbal IQ based on the Vocabulary, Digit Span and Similarities subtests is at least 10 IQ points lower than a prorated performance IQ based on the Block Design and Object Assembly subtests.

The prorating is accomplished as follows: for the prorated verbal IQ add the Vocabulary, Digit Span, and Similarities subtest scores, multiply by two and use the obtained value to find the IQ in the WAIS manual. For the prorated performance IQ add the Block Design and Object Assembly scores, multiply by 2.5 and again determine the IQ by looking up the obtained value in the WAIS manual.

B. Criterion for right hemisphere brain damage: The sum of all points lateralizing to the right hemisphere is at least twice as large as the sum of all points lateralizing to the left hemisphere. Indicators for right hemisphere brain damage:

1. Two-point indicators

a. The score for the Spatial Relations Test must be at least three rating points worse than the score for the Aphasia Test.

b. Right-handed people must average more than 20 fewer taps with their left hand than with their right. Left-handed people must average more than five fewer taps with their left hand than with their right.

2. One-point indicators
   a. The score for Spatial Relations Test must be one rating point poorer than the Aphasia Test score.
   b. TPT-Left Hand time score must be worse than TPT-Right Hand time score by at least two rating points.
   c. Average tapping speed. For right-handed people, more than 10 taps slower with the left hand than with the right. For left-handed people the tapping speed with the left hand must be slower than with the right.
   d. There must be more impairment of sensory function on the left side of the body than on the right. This indicator is said to be present if any *one* of the following are present:
      (1) At least 2.5 times as many errors are made on the Finger Agnosia Test with the left hand as with the right. (Invalid if there are less than four errors with the left hand.)
      (2) At least 2.5 times as many errors are made on the Finger-Tip Number Writing Test with the left hand as with the right. (Invalid if there are less than six errors with the left hand.)
      (3) The rating for hypesthesia of the left side must be at least 2.5 times that obtained for the right side. (Invalid if the rating for the left hand is less than three.)
   e. Suppression on double simultaneous stimulation must be more severe on the left side than on the right. This indicator is said to be present if any *one* of the following is true:
      (1) At least 2.5 as many suppressions of the left ear are made than of the right ear on double simultaneous auditory stimulation. (Invalid if there are less than three suppressions of the left ear.)
      (2) At least 2.5 times as many suppressions of tactual stimulation are made on the left side than on the right side on double simultaneous tactual stimulation. (Invalid if there are less than four suppressions on the left side.)
      (3) At least 2.5 times as many suppressions of the left visual field than of the right visual field must occur on double simultaneous visual stimulation. (Invalid if there are less than four suppressions of the left field.)

      NOTE: The note made concerning intactness of primary sensory functions appearing under the left hemisphere section of this key also obtains here.
   f. A left homonymous hemianopia is found. The same method as described for identifying right homonymous hemianopias is used here. (See II 2 f.)

g. On the WAIS there must be more impairment on the performance tests than on the verbal tests. This indicator is present if a prorated performance IQ based on the Block Design and Object Assembly subtests is at least 10 IQ points lower than a prorated verbal IQ based on the Vocabulary, Digit Span and Similarities subtests. The method of prorating is described in the section on the use of the WAIS in identifying left hemisphere brain damage. (See II 2 g.)

C. Criterion for diffuse brain damage: If brain damage has not been classified as lateralizing to either hemisphere, classify as diffuse.

B. The Degree of Lateralization Key

I. Establish the presence of left or right hemisphere brain damage using the Localization Key. (The present key is not to be used for cases classified as diffuse by the Localization Key.)

II. Criteria for strong lateralization:

A. At least one two-point indicator, lateralizing to the hemisphere indicated by the Localization Key, must be present.

B. There must be at least three more one-point indicators for the hemisphere indicated by the Localization Key than for the other hemisphere.

III. Criterion for weak lateralization:

A. All cases lateralized by the Localization Key, but not meeting the criteria stated in II A or II B above are classified as weakly lateralized.

C. The Process Key

I. Determine presence or absence of brain damage. Criterion: Average Impairment Rating is less than 1.55.

NO BRAIN DAMAGE—STOP

II. If brain damage is present (Average Impairment Rating equal to or greater than 1.55) determine process.

A. Criteria for acute brain damage:

1. Severe impairment must be present.

a. The Average Impairment Rating must be equal to or greater than three.

b. The Degree of Lateralization Key must classify the case as strongly lateralized to the right or left cerebral hemisphere.

ACUTE BRAIN DAMAGE—STOP

B. Criteria for congenital brain damage:

1. Classify as congenital brain damage if the Average Impairment Rating is less than three. The Key classifies the case as diffuse or weakly lateralized, and either of the following:

a. The WAIS full scale IQ is less than or equal to 98 and either mixed hand or crossed-eye dominance is present. (See Appendix E.)

b. The WAIS full scale IQ is less than or equal to 80 and either (1) or (2) below are true.
   (1) The average of the ratings for tapping and perceptual disorders is equal to or less than 1.5.
   (2) There is no more than a five-point discrepancy between WAIS verbal and performance IQs.

CONGENITAL BRAIN DAMAGE—STOP

C. Criterion for static brain damage:
   1. Neither A nor B above.

STATIC BRAIN DAMAGE—STOP

Three examples are given to illustrate how the Keys are applied. The first example includes all the aspects of the case evaluation used in this study, namely the Key results, the neuropsychological report and the neurological examinational findings. This information is presented in Appendix F. The other examples are limited to the application of the Keys.

Example 1. This is case number 180, a 56-year old man with a diagnosis of acoustic neuroma. The neuroma was surgically removed but the evaluation to be reported on here was done presurgically. The basic data on this subject are given in the abbreviated neurological interim summary in Appendix F and need not be repeated here. While the surgical intervention allowed for reasonably definite location of the site of the lesion, the neurological report only indicates that it was in the right occipital area of the brain. Acoustic neuromas start on the VIIIth cranial nerve and so may sometimes result only in the impairment of functions mediated by the brain stem. In this case, however, the presence of a left hemiparesis and positive pneumoencephalographic findings indicated involvement of the cerebral cortex and so the case was included in the total pool (Phase 1 of the procedure). The neurological assignments to the categories used by the Keys (Phase 2) were quite clear. They were right hemisphere lesion for the Localization Key and acute brain damage for the Process Key, since all rapidly progressive cerebral tumors were considered to be acute lesions.

The neuropsychological examination (Phase 3) was made less than 3 weeks after the patient entered the hospital. It was stated in the neuropsychological report (Appendix F) that the patient had a diffuse disease because there was bilateral involvement but that the right cerebral hemisphere was functioning more poorly than the left. The case was returned to the neuropsychologist who then categorized it into the right hemisphere lateralization category. The neuropsychological report also stated that the disease was active, probably a tumor. This statement, of course, places the case into the acute process category.

The keying procedure (Phase 4) was based on the results of the neuropsychological testing presented in the Neuropsychological Key summary sheet appearing in Appendix F, p. 123. This sheet contains all the scores that are needed to "run" the Key. Beginning with the Localization Key, we find that the Average Impairment Rating for this patient is 4.17, a score that greatly exceeds the score of 1.55 needed to classify the case as brain damaged. The next step is to determine lateralization. Here one must determine whether or not there are twice as many points lateralizing to one hemisphere as to the other. With regard to the left hemisphere two-point indicators, criteria for 1 a and b are not met. Spatial relations is worse than aphasia, and the patient's tapping speeds are the same for both hands. (The patient is right handed.) With regard to the one-point indicators of left hemisphere damage, the following criteria are and are not met:

II a 2 a is not met because the spatial relations test score is worse than the aphasia test score.

II a 2 b is not met because the time score for the TPT is the same for both hands. II a 2 c is not met because tapping speed is not slower with the right hand.

II a 2 d 1 is not met because there are not 2.5 times as many errors with the right hand as with the left. For the same reason, criteria for II a 2 d 2 and II a 2 d 3 are not met.

The criterion for II a 2 e 1 is not met because the test is invalid (presence of primary hearing loss rated 4). II a 2 e 2 and II a 2 e 3 are not met, nor is II a 2 f, since a right homonymous hemianopia was not found. II a 2 g is not met, since the prorated performance IQ is lower than the prorated verbal IQ. Thus, a total of 0 points for the left hemisphere is obtained.

With regard to the right hemisphere two-point indicators, the criterion for II B 1 a is met because the spatial relations test score is at least three points worse than the aphasia test score. The criterion for II B 1 b, however, is not met.

With regard to the 1-point indicators, the criterion for II B 2 a is met. The criterion for II B 2 b, c and d are not met. The criteria for II B 2 e 1 and 2 are not met, but criterion is met for II B 2 e 3 since there are 6 left visual field suppressions and only two right visual field suppressions. A left homonymous hemianopia was not found, and so the criterion for II B 2 f is not met. The criterion for II B 2 g is met because the prorated performance IQ is at least 10 points lower than the prorated verbal IQ. Thus a total of five points for the right hemisphere is found. Since the total of right hemisphere points (5) is at least twice as great as the total of left hemisphere points (0), the case is placed into the right hemisphere brain damage category.

Since a lateralization was established, the Degree of Lateralization Key is used. The criterion stated under II A of that key is met, and so the case goes into the strongly lateralized to the right hemisphere category.

Proceeding to the Process Key, the presence of brain damage is again established, since the Average Impairment Rating is greater than 1.55.

Since an Average Impairment Rating greater than three was found, as were indications of strong lateralization, the criteria set forth under II A 1 a and b are met. Thus, the case is placed into the acute brain damage category. Combining the Keys, it can be said that the patient has acute brain damage, the lesion being strongly lateralized to the right cerebral hemisphere. Inspection of Appendix H, Case 180, indicates that the case was classified similarly by the neurologist and the neuropsychologist.

Example 2. Case number 154 is the second example. The Key summary sheet may be found in Appendix G. The Average Impairment Rating for this patient is 1.25. Since this score is lower than 1.55, the case is placed into the "no brain damage" category and no further application of any of the keys is required. This case is presented simply to illustrate the point that use of the Key is terminated in all cases in which there is an Average Impairment Rating of less than 1.55.

Example 3. Case number 464 will be used for the third example. The Neuropsychological Key summary may be found in Appendix G. Starting again with the Localization Key, the *S*s Average Impairment Rating of 2.83 meets the criterion for placement into the brain damaged category. Neither of the criteria for the two-point left-hemisphere indicators are met. The ratings for the aphasia and spatial relations tests are equal, and he does not tap more slowly with his right hand than with his left. He is right handed. With regard to the one-point left-hemisphere indicators, only II A 2 d 1 meets criterion. On the Finger Agnosia Test he makes 2.5 times as many errors with his right hand as with his left. No points are earned on the right hemisphere indicators. Since there are less than twice as many points lateralizing to one hemisphere as compared with the other hemisphere (1 point for the left hemisphere and nine points for the right hemisphere) the case is classified as "diffuse brain damage" by process of elimination.

Since the lesion was not lateralized, the Degree of Lateralization Key is not applicable here. Proceeding with the Process Key, the presence of brain damage is again established on the basis of the Average Impairment Rating. Neither of the acute brain damage criteria are met. The patient's Average Impairment Rating is less than three and he does not have strong lateralizing signs. It is necessary to proceed to II B, the congenital brain damage category. Both criteria for II B 1 are met; the Average Impairment Rating is less than three and the Localization Key Classified the case as diffuse. The criterion for II B 1 a is also met, since the WAIS full scale IQ is less than 98, and the patient has crossed hand-eye dominance. The use of the Process Key is terminated at this point, and the case is classified into the congenital brain damage category. Combining the results of all keys, it can be said that the patient has diffuse, congenital brain damage.

CHAPTER 5

The Neurological Criterion for Keys

Perhaps the major problem that the neuropsychologist must deal with is the validity of his criterion. There are many excellent general discussions of this subject in the literature (Hebb, 1949; Meyer, 1961; Reitan, 1962). Consequently the general problem will only be handled briefly as an introduction to the specific criterion problems that were dealt with in the development of the current neuropsychological keys.

Perhaps one of the reasons that the criterion problem has been so thoroughly investigated in relation to brain damage is that unlike many areas of psychology a concrete, objective criterion exists. Thus the problems of determining validity can be examined meaningfully. Although the criteria are often difficult to determine in human brain damage studies, a comparison of them to the usual criteria used in most clinical psychology research, for instance MMPI studies (Dahlstrom and Welsh, 1960), indicates how good the brain damage criteria are—relatively speaking.

GENERAL PROBLEM

The ideal criterion for human brain damage research is that used in animal studies. In these studies not only is the lesion placed with fair precision in an otherwise normal animal but also the animal's brain is examined after the completion of the experiment to determine the exact extent and location of the lesion. For obvious reasons such procedures cannot be used in humans. Here the lesion is generally produced by chance factors and even when surgically produced the location is determined by therapeutic requirements that have no relationship to research except through accident. At times, as in much of Penfield's work (1966), the research is designed to conform to the lesion being made rather than the lesion being placed to conform to the research requirements.

Reitan (1962) indicates some of the methods by which various investigators of human brain damage have attempted to increase the accuracy of the criterion. Most of these investigators have done this by selecting certain types of brain damaged cases with considerable care. The work in Teuber's laboratory has concentrated on studying residual effects of relatively old brain injuries. The attempt is to locate the injury accurately (these were often penetrating head injuries) and use the same patients in many studies (Teuber, 1962). Milner (1956, 1962) has worked on pre- and postoperative cases. Talland (1963) even restricted his population to cases of Korsakoff's psychosis.

If the patient population is sufficiently large, selection can begin to isolate the lesion within the brain though this can never approach the accuracy of animal research. The need for this selection creates several new problems not found in animal studies.

First, to select cases of a particular kind requires a very large population from which to obtain these cases. The result is that, usually, studies use relatively small numbers of subjects drawn from a huge pool of cases. Since brain damage is not particularly common in our society, the laboratories must be located in large population centers (Teuber uses all of New York City) and the time to collect cases may be considerable. Reitan (1964a) took several years to collect four good cases limited to each quarter of the brain.

Reitan and his students adopted one method of overcoming this difficulty (Reitan, 1966). A battery of tests were administered without variation over several years and a large pool of cases was thus created from which the desired categories could be selected. This approach was also used in this study. The entire pool of cases collected in Goldstein's laboratory over a three-year period was utilized even though in this study the categories utilized were fairly general and common. Nevertheless, several aspects of this study originally under consideration had to be abandoned due to a lack of appropriate cases.

A second problem that is usually a complicating factor and that requires large samples to be used even though these are hard to obtain is that pre- and posttesting is seldom possible with humans. Weinstein and Teuber (1957) attempted to make use of this procedure a number of years ago by readministering the Army General Classification Test to soldiers who had been brain injured in the war. Here the difficulty was that the AGCT was not designed to test brain damage. As a result it evidently picked up only the verbal difficulties related to the left hemisphere (Reitan, 1962).

There have been attempts to give pre- and posttesting to patients who have cerebral operations. There was a rash of studies on lobotomy patients done in the early 1950's. The results of these studies like that of the Columbia-Greystone studies (Mettler, 1949, 1952) were discouraging with regard to their contribution to our knowledge of brain localization. In part this was due to the use of poor experimental designs (Mettler, 1952) but it was also due to the condition that almost all the operations were done on patients with severe preexisting psychoses. This introduced deficits in the subject's performance that could not be separated from the results of the lobotomy.

Such difficulties have also been true for the studies on patients who had ablation of parts of their cortex in order to control epileptogenic scar tissue (Milner, 1962). Hebb (1949) has pointed out the effect an epileptogenic scar formation may have on brain functioning. Thus the results of pre- and posttesting may be due not only to the effect of the operation but to a preexisting abnormality. The results of such preexisting abnormalities were very evident in some of the research done under Sperry (1961). Three cases of humans who had their cerebral commissures sectioned in order to relieve epilepsy were thoroughly tested. The results obtained were not equivalent. The reason for this subsequently appeared to be that the earliest case tested had sustained some lateralized brain damage prior to the commissurotomy and this was sufficient to disrupt the results of psychological testing. Thus the latter two cases, which were more intact prior to the operation, produced different results on the psychological testing (Gazzaniga & Sperry, 1967). The conclusions from testing the first case were evidently somewhat erroneous from the point of view of normal brain functioning.

NEUROLOGICAL EXAMINATION AS A CRITERION FOR BRAIN DAMAGE KEYS

In spite of these secondary difficulties in selecting cases for a criterion of types of brain damage, the major problem is still to obtain an adequate neurological diagnosis. There are many difficulties in this area, of which the neurologists are well aware. Neurological reports vary in their probable accuracy depending on several factors. First, the neurologist's report may not offer the information that the neuropsychological researcher desires. The standard or physical neurological examination is designed to determine what kind of disease process exists in the patient and the type of therapeutic procedure to recommend. Consequently, certain types of investigative procedures are not always utilized, such as angiograms, since they are not always warranted and may be dangerous or costly. Unfortunately from the point of view of neuropsychology research (but not from that of the patient's welfare), the most accurate procedures for diagnosing the extent and location of brain damage are operative procedures which are not routinely utilized.

There is a hierarchy of procedures in neurological practice which becomes more accurate as it is ascended. At the bottom of the hierarchy is the physical neurological examination which is the least accurate. Its validity depends upon a tradition of gradually accumulating knowledge derived from the procedures higher in the hierarchy. The higher procedures involve more direct examination of the brain itself. At the top of the hierarchy are the autopsy and the brain operation, in which case the brain is directly observed.

Next in order are the operative procedures which involve a semiobservation of the brain and require minor surgical procedures. These are the pneumoencephalograph and angiograms. Next are procedures that are not operative but require special equipment and techniques such as the electroencephalograph and the brain scan. Finally the neurological examination at the bottom derives its validity from the procedures higher on the scale. This, however, does not mean it is not very valid. Rather it only means that its validity is dependent on the other procedures higher in the scale. However, in actual practice the higher on the scale one ascends the less often is the procedure used because it involves greater risk to the patient's life and comfort. In this study which used 106 subjects the number of cases in which operative procedures were used was quite small and only one autopsy was contributory.

Even the highest procedures on the hierarchy have weaknesses as far as being a validating criterion is concerned. By analogy with animal research an autopsy examination might be considered to be the best criterion for brain damage research. However, there are several problems here. First, patients tend to live on indefinitely (Hebb, 1949) so autopsy can seldom be extensively utilized except for certain conditions, such as tumors and other illnesses in which the patient dies shortly after acquisition of the lesion. The nature of these conditions themselves, however, often reduce the utility of the autopsy. Tumor patients cannot be tested after the tumor has become extensive and since tumors grow and infiltrate it is often impossible to determine the area or even the location of the brain lesion which the subject had at the time of testing from the post-mortem examination (Reitan, 1966).

Each of the other procedures have their particular form of difficulty as a criterion. In an operation one's vision is generally limited so that the location in the brain may not be exactly determined (Mettler, 1949). Generally, a postoperative examination of the excised tissue is necessary in order to determine exactly what part of the brain was removed and even this procedure is not always definitive.

The primary difficulties of the other procedures, such as pneumoencephalography and angiography, are that they will not demonstrate all forms of brain damage. Each has advantages and limitations which need not be discussed here.

There are several modifying circumstances that improve this situation. First, the total neurological examination usually makes use of enough of the necessary procedures to make a valid diagnosis. The number of procedures necessary depends on the particular case. Cases whose validity cannot be determined because of missing information can often be eliminated from the sample as they have been in this study.

Second, the precision of the validity required varies in relation to the kind of study being made. Thus the type of information available varies in validity and the type required by a study varies. The validity of a criterion need not be perfect. It must simply be sufficient for the purposes of the study being made. Consequently the next section attempts to evaluate the criterion used for this study.

NEUROLOGICAL CRITERION USED IN THIS STUDY

In regard to criterion problems that were specific to this study, the first involved the use of the physical neurological examination report. In all brain damage studies the neurologist's report must remain the basic criterion. The question is whether the report from the usual physical examination can be used as an adequate criterion. Most of the reports used in this study utilized procedures which were rather low in the criterion validity hierarchy previously described. Although the validity of these reports cannot be numerically determined, they were supervised by Dr. D. B. Foster and Dr. J. Stein of the staff of the Menninger Foundation who are both experienced, board certified neurologists.

Validity of the Neurological Examination

Essentially the validity of the neurological examination was not primarily relevant to this study. The primary purpose of this study was not to determine whether a certain test assesses the actual existence of certain types of brain damage but whether it would predict or agree with the neurological examination. That is, the validity of the neurological examination was not in question, but assumed. The validity question simply concerned how well the key could duplicate the neuropsychological examination in predicting the results of the neurological examination.

In this regard one might wish to distinguish between two kinds of validity. In one kind the actual neurological disease process serves as criterion. This type is certainly a highly desirable one, and it can be accomplished in those cases in which site and type of lesion can be precisely determined. The other kind of validation utilizes an independent procedure as the criterion, and while not as desirable as the first type, it must be resorted to in cases in which direct specification of type and site cannot be accomplished. In the present study this second type of validation was used because of the difficulties inherent in the direct specification of type and locus of brain lesions in humans. However, since neuropsychological testing and the neurological examination are independent procedures, one can be validated against the other. The obvious difficulty with this method is that in some unknown proportion of the cases studied, the criterion may be in error; that is, the neurological examination may lead to an erroneous diagnosis. When this is the case, and the neuropsychological methods make the same error, there is agreement and the accuracy of the neuropsychological method is spuriously inflated. When there is disagreement, however, the neuropsychological method may have predicted the correct diagnosis, but its accuracy may be spuriously deflated because the prediction did not agree with the erroneous one made on the basis of the neurological examination. Because of the relatively primitive state of neurological diagnosis of brain lesions, the neuropsychologist interested in the study of humans must live with these difficulties. Studies relating neuropsychological test findings to neurological criteria may have a mutual "bootstrap" effect in that if the same conclusions can be reached in a preponderance of cases by the independent and different methods of the neuropsychologist and the neurologist, it becomes increasingly likely that both methods have accurately predicted the objective situation (i.e., the actual neurological disease process). In essence it is maintained that accuracy of prediction is increased as the number of independent methods making the same prediction is increased.

Validity of the Neuropsychological Examination

The problem of determining the validity of the neuropsychological examination as a criterion for the Key was somewhat different from examining the validity of the neurological examination. In this case, since the Key and the neuropsychological examination utilize the same tests and measures in their analysis, the agreement between these methods was not related to the neurological validity of either one. Their agreement, rather, indicated how closely the Key had objectified the implicit logic and criteria used by the neuropsychologist. The agreement between the Key and the neuropsychologist's report was probably only limited by the inherent variability or reliability in the inferential method (Meehl, 1959).

In addition, the validity of the neuropsychological examination can be determined by comparing its results to the results of the neurological report. This was done for the Localization Key in Tables 7 and 15. These tables demonstrate that the neuropsychological examination agrees with the neurological with a significance beyond the .001 level. The ability of the neuropsychologist to predict the neurological examination results for individual categories in terms of percent of the neurological cases correctly predicted varies from 73 to 92 (Tables 12 and 20). From these results the neuropsychological examination appears to be highly valid and so can legitimately be a criterion for the Key.

To summarize, in this study the validity of the neurological examination was simply assumed when it was utilized as the final criterion. This, of course, was also true in regard to the neuropsychological report when it was utilized as the criterion. However, a measure of its agreement with the neurological was obtained which demonstrated its validity. The Key, in any case, was designed not to predict the "real" nature of the brain damage but rather to predict the neurological examination and to objectify the neuropsychological examination. Statistical measures of agreement under these conditions were utilized to determine the Key's validity. Eventually, of course, Keys may be designed and validated against only the most reliable neurological procedures. Under these conditions their validity would hopefully be improved or at least be more accurately established.

CHAPTER 6

Method of Validation, Part I: Neurological Selection

GENERAL PROCEDURE

The purpose of this research study, discussed earlier in a general way, can be made more explicit here. Under certain conditions, such as determining the type of brain damage that affects a person, the inferential method ("clinical intuition") can produce more accurate results than can actuarial methods (Reitan, 1964a). In spite of its being inferential, Reitan thought that the necessary information was available to the neuropsychologists who made the evaluations. The problem was to create an objective method that would duplicate the inferential process and utilize that information. The primary purpose of this study was to create and validate such an objective method.

The method selected constituted an adaptation of the biological Key method. The two Keys created are described in Chapter 3. The remaining problem was to validate these Keys.

The method of validation was that of criterion validation in which the Keys were compared to two kinds of criteria. Since the Key was designed to duplicate the neuropsychologist's inferential process, the first criterion was the neuropsychological examination results as given in the neuropsychological reports. The second criterion was the one utilized to validate the neuropsychological results themselves, that is, the neurological examination findings. Thus in the second method of validation the Keys' results were compared against the neurological examination.

There were several other purposes that have guided the form of the study. First a Key such as this has several practical advantages. It enables a relatively unskilled person to make the classifications that now require the labor of a highly trained neuropsychologist. As can be seen in the Appendices, the Key can be read with a computer, making for even greater simplification in interpreting neurological data.

Summary of Method Procedure

In order to clarify the method of validation the total procedure can be summarized in terms of five phases. The first phase consisted of the selection of cases from the files to produce a total pool of 106 cases which included 26 controls.

Phase 2 consisted of using the neurological examination to sort the total pool of cases into the categories used by the two Keys. This created one pool of subjects for each Key, a localization pool and a process pool. A subject from the total pool could be placed in both pools if the case met the relevant criteria. These two phases are dealt with in detail later in this chapter in the sections entitled "Selection of Cases" and "Interpretation of Neurological Diagnosis."

Phase 3 used the neuropsychological reports to classify the subjects for each pool into the Key categories. This phase was accomplished without reference to Phase 2. This procedure eliminated a few additional cases in the process pool so that the final process pool contained 73 subjects (22 controls) and the localization pool contained 104 cases (26 controls).

Phase 4, again accomplished independently, utilized a clerk, who had no formal knowledge of brain damage, to apply the Keys to the neuropsychological raw data.

Phase 5 consisted of a statistical comparison of the results from the neurological reports, the neuropsychological inferential reports and the Keys. The details of these phases are given in Chapters 5, 6, and 8.

Description of the Neuropsychological Laboratory

Before the selection criteria can be explained, a short account of the nature of the Topeka Veterans Administration Hospital neurological service and neuropsychological laboratory needs to be given. This volume was written utilizing material from the neuropsychological laboratory in this hospital which is under the direction of Dr. Goldstein.

The Topeka Veterans Administration Hospital is principally a neuropsychiatric hospital although one section comprises a medium size general hospital with a neurology floor. Patients were referred to the neuropsychological laboratory from all parts of the hospital although most of the referrals came from the Neurology Service. This hospital has a close relationship with the nearby Menninger Foundation; consequently many staff members work or consult in both institutions. This was the case with the neurologist D. B. Foster, who supervised most of the neurological examinations used as the criteria for this study. The neuropsychologist P. M. Rennick, mentioned earlier, was on the staff of the Menninger Foundation while G. Goldstein was on the staff of the Topeka Veterans Administration Hospital. However, they worked together closely after Rennick had introduced Goldstein to the neuropsychological laboratory procedures. The neuropsychological laboratory at the Topeka Veterans Administration Hospital was part of the research division of this hospital which was under the supervision of a psychologist, J. W. Chotlos. Many other kinds of research were also in process.

There was a fairly close relationship between the neuropsychological laboratory and the Neurology Service. All neurological patients able to take the Halstead-Reitan Battery were referred automatically to the neuropsychological laboratory. Usually this was after they had been given neurological examinations. Also, copies of all neurological examination and case summary reports from the Neurology Service were sent to the neuropsychological laboratory. The neuropsychological reports were written by Goldstein who had neither seen the patient nor been given any information about him except the test scores and his age, occupation and education. It was only after the neuropsychological report had been completed that the neurological report was read and placed in the files. Thus the inferential neuropsychological report and the neurological report were written separately and without reference to each other. There were a few cases in which this separation was not complete; these "contaminated" cases were removed and not used in this study.

SELECTION OF CASES

The first difficulty which arose in this study was the correct selection of cases (from the files) on which to apply the Key (Phase 1 of the procedure). The files contained every kind of case that might come to the attention of the Neurology Service including both brain damaged cases and suspected brain damage cases. The Key was not constructed to handle all kinds of "neurological" cases but only those with cortical damage uncomplicated by peripheral damage or severe emotional factors. The subjects used in this study were thus limited to a certain group of cases. However, this group was broad and essentially it consisted of all cases which could be adequately tested by the neuropsychological examination.

Fundamentally, four kinds of cases were eliminated. (The selective procedure is given in Chapter 7 under "Subject Population.") These were cases in which peripheral damage interfered with the test results; that is, if a subject had only one arm, the tests in the battery that compare right and left hands could not be utilized. In many cases the neuropsychologist can adjust to this situation in order to write his report but the Key as now constructed cannot do so. The second general reason for elimination of cases is that the effects of certain functional difficulties such as hysteria or schizophrenia are not known and so they could not be taken into consideration by the Key. The third general reason for eliminating cases was that the neurological examination was not sufficiently adequate to determine the category into which the cases should be placed. If for some reason no neurological report was available, that case could not be utilized. The fourth reason was contamination of the neurological report by the neuropsychological report. Most neurological reports were made independently of the results of the neuropsychological report; however, in a few cases the neuropsychological report was used to determine the neurological diagnosis. Such cases were considered to be contaminated.

Table 1. Selection Criteria

Reason for Elimination	N
1. Peripheral damage	12
2. Peripheral neurological disease	5
3. Acute brain syndrome	6
4. Schizophrenia	12
5. Somaticizing neurosis	7
6. Incomplete neurological	32
7. Diagnosis complex	19
8. Contamination	5
Total	98
Reason for Elimination: Process Key Only *	
1. Diagnosis complex	15
2. Trauma occurred between 3 months and 1 year prior to testing	7
3. Incomplete neuropsychological	11
Total	33

* Two cases were acceptable for the Process Key that were not for Localization Key. They both had multiple areas of damage.

Table 1 gives a more complete breakdown of the specific criteria used to eliminate cases and the number of cases eliminated for each reason. The second part of the table states reasons utilized to eliminate cases that would not fit the process key. These are in addition to the general reasons given at the top of the table.

Some of the reasons in Table 1 are self-explanatory while others need a short explanation or elaboration. The category called "peripheral damage" was largely self-explanatory while neurological disease needs some explanation. Peripheral neurological diseases, such as myasthenia gravis, will affect parts of the brain damage battery, such as tapping speed, although they do not affect cortical functioning. Multiple sclerosis generally begins with noncortical dysfunction and then progresses to the brain and cortex. Thus at different times it is both a noncortical and a cortical disease. For this reason early cases were eliminated while older cases with several hospitalizations were assumed to involve cortical damage and were retained in the total pool.

Acute brain syndromes, schizophrenia and somaticizing neurosis may all affect the brain damage battery although permanent cortical damage is not present; consequently they were eliminated. Somaticizing neurosis included the kinds of neurosis in which the symptoms may affect the brain damage battery to any great extent. Thus conversion reactions were eliminated while anxiety reactions without major somatic complications were retained and became part of the control group.

Most of the cases listed under "incomplete neurological" were missing report protocols. During one short period the neurological department did not routinely send a copy of the neurological report to the research department so these case files contain no neurological report. The bulk of the cases in this category belong to this period.

The most common reason for a "complex diagnosis" was that the etiology was unknown. The other major reason was that a mixture of diagnoses prevented exact categorization. Both of the cases that could be handled by the Process Key and not by the Localization Key were of this nature. Of the cases included in the pool, 17 had multiple diagnoses. However, they either had a primary diagnosis of brain damage or the effects of the alternative diagnosis were not such as to prevent the case from being included in the pool.

Thirty-three cases in the total pool could not be used for the Process Key. The general reasons for their elimination are also given in Table 1. "Diagnosis complex" included such cases as those which had two kinds of brain damage so that they were both acute and static. Here probably the largest group was arteriosclerotic patients with mild cerebral vascular accidents. One is acute, the other static. If the accident was severe, the acute effects were assumed to dominate the static effects so the case was categorized as acute. An old cerebral vascular accident was, of course, classed as static.

If the trauma occurred three months to one year before testing, the case was eliminated, since it did not fit the definition for either acute (three months old or less) or static process (more than a year old).

The final category of reasons for eliminating cases for the process pool was related to the mechanics of this research. Cases were initially selected on the basis of the neurological report. However, when the neuropsychological report was inspected for the process category assessment, 11 protocols either did not indicate the stage of process or used a term which indicated an intermediate category between the acute and static stage. The key could not handle such cases, so they were rejected. Since certain types of patients were eliminated from the study, the reader who wishes to make use of the Keys with these patients should do so with caution.

INTERPRETATION OF NEUROLOGICAL DIAGNOSIS

The last major difficulty in selecting the criterion cases was to determine into which category the neurological report placed a case (Phase 2 of the procedure). The neurological reports seldom directly state the kind of information needed to place a subject into the categories that were utilized by the Keys. This was especially true of the Localization Key. The "official" diagnosis does not contain a localization statement. The nearest to such a statement wculd be a diagnosis such as "cerebral thrombosis with a right hemiplegia." This, of course, required translation into left-sided brain damage.

Other cases required interpretation of the neurological examination by reference to either the neurological results, the case history or the diagnosis. Often the neurological report would mention that one side of the body contained more signs of deficit than the other. If not, the psychologist, through examining the report, had to make a judgment based on the reported neurological results; for instance, certain diagnostic categories such as alcoholic encephalopathy were routinely categorized as diffuse.

These judgments were made prior to and without reference to the neuropsychological report. However, in order to determine their reliability a group of 24 cases selected as the most difficult to classify in the localization pool were independently reclassified by G. Goldstein. There were five disagreements and 19 agreements (71% agreement). This level of agreement is not as high as might be desired, but is not so low as to vitiate the results of the study. An indirect indication of the reliability of these judgments was the final level of agreement between the Key and the neurological (Table 9). Since these two procedures were scored independently, the high level of agreement implies high reliability in understanding the intent of the neurologists' formulation of the case.

The situation in regard to the translation of the neurological report into the process categories was more direct and therefore more accurate.

The definitions of types of brain damage processes determined the criteria utilized in their selection. Acute brain damage was considered to be any brain damage which had occurred within three months of testing or a rapid progressive condition. A rapidly progressive condition was determined by the kind of diagnosis given to the case. Static brain damage was any kind of brain damage whose active stage had ceased for over a year or one in which there was at most a slowly progressive condition. This latter condition was also established by diagnosis. Although by definition congenital brain damage only includes damage that occurs during pregnancy or at birth, damage that occurred in infancy has similar neurological results so these cases were also included under the category of congenital brain damage. In this study a neurological diagnosis of congenital encephalopathy was used as the criterion. The case history was usually ambivalent in regard to the length of time the brain dysfunction had lasted. The acute category was quite specific. It contained obviously acute processes such as a tumor or recent trauma which could be dated. The congenital category was also fairly specific, at least in regard to the symptoms that indicated it. The static category contained almost everything else. The results of this difference in reliability can be observed in Tables 18 and 19.

The interpretation of the neuropsychological report was generally straightforward. The categories required were usually given directly in the report. A localization classification was always given and a process classification was usually given. In regard to process when it was not stated, that case was eliminated from the process pool.

The only major difficulty encountered in scoring the neuropsychological report was that it often gave a mixed classification such as, "This is a diffuse process with maximal involvement in the right hemisphere," or "The left hemisphere is most damaged although diffuse effects are evident."

The test battery enabled the neuropsychologist to make such mixed judgments, but the Key required a definite categorization. This difficulty was handled by having the author of the neuropsychological reports, Dr. Goldstein, reevaluate the test results and categorize the subjects. Dr. Goldstein was not aware of the neurological diagnoses or of the Key categorizations. Thus his judgments could not be influenced by knowledge of the conclusions made by the Key or by the neurologist.

CHAPTER 7

Method of Validation, Part II: Neuropsychological Operations

SUBJECT POPULATION

Initial Selection

The subject cases for this research were selected from the neuropsychology files at the Topeka Veterans Administration Hospital (Phase 1). All cases in the file that were complete and were available from case number 150 to 663 were utilized. Completed cases are ones in which the neuropsychological testing had been done and the neuropsychological report had been written. Most of these cases also contained the report of the neurological examination along with a case history. The existence of a neurological report, however, was not a factor in the first selection. In addition, about 12 cases that had evidently been completed could not be located and constituted the cases that were not available.

The cases utilized began at case number 150 due to both the general lack of neurological reports before that number and the fact that the early cases had been utilized for initial studies on this Key. The cases utilized were all the cases from number 150 to the time that the selection of cases was begun. The last case tested prior to this time was case number 663. Thus all complete and available cases tested in the neuropsychological laboratory between August 1965 to July 1967 were used. This constituted almost the entire output of two years of neuropsychological testing. During most of this time two full-time testers were employed.

The number of cases initially utilized was 204. Since a conservative estimate was that at least 12 hours of testing went into each case this constituted 2448 hours of testing. In this group of 204 cases 98 were eliminated using criteria listed in Table 1 leaving 106 cases that constituted the total pool of cases utilized in this study. The Localization Key could be applied to all but two of the total pool cases making the localization sample 104 cases. The cases that could fit the requirements for the Process Key were fewer in number. There were 73 cases in the process sample. The specific criteria for selecting cases is discussed in Chapter 6 and complete data for each subject in the total pool are given in Appendix H.

Controls

There was no initial attempt to select controls since a number of cases had been sent to the neuropsychological laboratory for testing that had both a negative neurological and a negative history. It should be noted, however, that in all of these cases there was some suspicion of brain damage and a referral for neuropsychological examination was made in order to disconfirm this suspicion. Thus some of these cases may have had mild amounts of brain damage that could not be definitely demonstrated by the standard physical neurological examination. The total number of controls was 26 or about one-fourth of the cases in the total pool.

Sources of Cases

The subjects for neuropsychological testing were referred to the laboratory from regular medical referral channels. There was an attempt to test all cases handled by the Neurological Service which were testable. The rest of the cases were referred by other sections of the hospital. However, only part of these cases were actually tested since the waiting period was often long and patients were discharged before they could be evaluated. Some of the cases that were "interesting" or that were referred on a priority basis were taken out of order. In spite of these factors the pool of cases evidently forms a rather typical cross section of male neurological cases found in any neuropsychiatric hospital.

Even though this was a veterans' hospital the number of injuries that were caused by particularly military hazards was minimal. Only one case in the total pool had brain damage due to a combat injury and two others were injured initially by explosions during military training.

Sex, Race, and Religion

In regard to the kind of data necessary to evaluate the results of a brain damage study experience with brain damage testing indicated that neither sex, nor race, nor religion could contribute any information that was not better given under other categories. Since this was a veterans' hospital only two women were tested as is indicated in Table 2. The race and religion of subjects were not recorded.

Age

The age of subjects was a potential source of influence on the results of this study. The statistical description of the various groups used in this

Table 2. Age and Sex of Subjects

Group	N	Mean	S.D.	Range	No. of Females
Total pool	106	46.07	14.26	19–79	2
Localization	104	45.85	14.25	19–79	2
Process	73	46.48	12.45	24–79	2
Controls (total)	26	44.54 *	13.07	24–79	0

* The difference between controls and the other groups was not significant at .05 level using Student's *t* test.

study is given in Table 2. The mean age for the total pool was 46.07 years and the other groups, including the control group, do not deviate much from this figure. The range and standard deviation demonstrated that this group was quite well age distributed and was not particularly loaded with older age subjects as might have been expected since many forms of brain damage are associated with aging. The relatively low number of veterans who would now be in the older age range probably accounts for this effect in part.

Although the mean age of the controls was a few years younger than the brain damaged group's, the standard deviations were so great that these differences did not approach significance using Student's *t*-test.

Intelligence

Although the intelligence of subjects is usually a crucial factor in evaluating the groups used in research it can only be used with great caution here since brain damage affects measured IQ. As part of the test battery all subjects were given the full WAIS and the results for various groups are recorded in Table 3. In this table the data are recorded for each of the three pools of subjects; total pool, localization pool and process pool. The controls are included in the pools, so that to compare the controls with the brain damaged subjects the controls were separated into the localization controls and process controls. The subjects left in the pools are the brain damaged subjects. They are designated as "localization brain damaged *S*s" and "process brain damaged *S*s". The difference between both the localization and process brain damaged groups and their controls was significant far beyond the .001 level, using Student's *t*-test. This is demonstrated in the lower section of Table 3.

The difference was probably due to the effect of brain damage since other studies have demonstrated such a decremental effect of brain damage (Reitan, 1960, Wechsler, 1944). In this case there were over 18 IQ points between the controls and brain damaged *S*s in both groups.

Table 3. WAIS Full Scale IQ of Subjects

Group	N	Mean	S.D.	Range
Total pool	106	95.91	14.66	63–133
Localization pool	104	95.85	14.77	63–133
Localization brain damaged Ss	78	91.27	12.76	63–119
Localization controls	26	109.58	11.52	93–133
Process pool	73	96.52	14.84	63–129
Process brain damaged Ss	51	90.98	12.65	63–112
Process controls	22	109.36	11.11	93–129

Tests of Significance

Group	t	df	Difference (IQ Points)
Localization brain damaged Ss versus controls	6.73 *	102	18.31
Process brain damaged Ss versus controls	6.11 *	71	18.38

* $P < .001$.

Since IQ measures obtained from the brain damaged subjects prior to acquisition of their brain lesions were not available to the authors, they have no direct way of estimating the premorbid IQ of these subjects. The alternative method commonly used to arrive at this estimate involves the use of tests known to be relatively insensitive to brain damage. Vocabulary tests of various sorts are often used for this purpose, and this procedure was the one chosen for the present study. All of the subjects received the WAIS, which has a vocabulary subtest. This method is not very satisfactory, particularly because a number of the brain damaged subjects in the present study had left hemisphere lesions. Lesions in this half of the brain are often associated with language dysfunction, and such dysfunction may impair vocabulary test performance substantially. However, no other means was available to assess premorbid level. The mean WAIS Vocabulary Subtest score for the subjects with neurologically documented brain lesions was 9.26 (S.D. = 2.52). The nonbrain damaged subjects obtained a mean score of 12.17 (S.D. = 2.85). A t test comparison yielded a t value of 4.76 ($p < .01$). These results support the hypothesis that the level of intellectual functioning of the control group is higher than the premorbid level of the brain damaged group. This finding is not surprising because verbal skills are affected by left hemisphere brain damage. There were also a number of individuals with congenital brain lesions in the brain damaged group and below average vocabularies are to be expected in this population. There is still some doubt that vocabulary tests yield an estimate of the premorbid level. In our own laboratory we have tested a number of patients before and after neurosurgery, and have found substantial improvement in vocabulary level on the post-surgery evaluation. Despite these questions about the adequacy of vocabulary as a measure of prebrain damage functioning the control group may well have had a somewhat higher level of functioning than did the brain damaged group premorbidly. The control group received more education than the brain damaged group, and since education and IQ are frequently found to be correlated, the view that the control group tended to have greater intellectual endowment than the brain damaged group is supported.

Education and Occupation

Education and level of occupation are often used in neuropsychology as rough measures of premorbid intelligence. The range of occupations included all levels of employment from unskilled labor to medical doctors. The percent of subjects at each occupational level gave an indication of the distribution. Although recorded, the occupations of the subjects were difficult to evaluate numerically. On the other hand, years of education gives a numerical measure and generally the amount of education and level of occupational skill appear to be strongly related.

The education of the subjects in years is given in Table 4. The mean for

Table 4. Education of Subjects in Years

Group	N	Mean	S.D.	Range
Total pool	106	11.45	3.30	4–23
Localization pool	104	11.46	3.31	4–23
Localization brain damaged Ss	78	11.05	3.68	4–23
Localization controls	26	12.69	3.35	7–21
Process pool	73	11.48	3.41	4–23
Process brain damaged Ss	51	10.88	3.24	4–23
Process controls	22	12.86	3.41	7–21

Tests of Significance

Group	t	df	Difference (years education)
Localization brain damaged Ss versus controls	2.08 *	102	1.64
Process brain damaged Ss versus controls	2.27 *	71	1.98

* $P < .05$.

the total pool was 11.45 which was just under the high school level of 12 years. The control groups had a small but statistically significant higher level of education than the brain damaged group. The mean difference between the controls and the brain damaged subjects in the localization pool was 1.64 years. This difference is significant at the .05 level using Student's *t* (Table 4). The difference between the controls and process pool patients was 1.98 years which also reached the .05 level of significance (Table 4).

The reason for this difference was difficult to determine. The removal of congenital brain damaged subjects who probably had a somewhat lower level of education did not raise the educational level of the brain damaged subjects sufficiently to account for much of the difference found.

Although this difference in education probably reflects a premorbid level of functioning higher for the controls than for the brain damaged subjects, it certainly could not account for the large IQ difference between the controls and brain damaged subjects.

In conclusion there appears to be a small but definite difference in the educational level between the controls and the brain damaged subjects for all the pools. This may indicate a difference in premorbid intelligence. This difference, however, was evidently not sufficient to have affected the results of this research. The Keys did not utilize the Full Scale IQ except as an indicator of congenital brain damage. Therefore it made only a minimal contribution to the overall classification process. Second, as has been indicated above, intelligence test performance in studies having to do with the effects of brain lesions on behavior can often be logically considered as a dependent variable; that is, there is a great deal of evidence (reviewed in Reitan, 1966) that brain damage may affect the measured IQ. In studies comparing brain damaged with nonbrain damaged control subjects, matching for IQ may be a questionable procedure in that it may produce a sample of brain damaged subjects who are natively brighter than their matched controls, but who have had their measured IQ reduced as a consequence of the brain damage. If one accepts this line of reasoning, matching subjects for IQ can create as many problems as it solves.

Diagnosis

The neurological diagnosis for each of the cases included in the total pool is given in Table 5. The number of cases in each diagnostic category for each of the groups utilized in this study is also tabulated. An examination of this table will reveal the wide range of diagnoses. This range is fairly representative of "run of the mill" neurological cases. Only two of the 21 categories contained more than 10 cases (controls were considered to be one category) and only seven categories had more than five cases.

Table 5. Diagnostic Categories of Subjects Giving the Number of Cases in Each Category for Each Subject Pool

Diagnosis of Brain Damage	Total	Location	Process
Trauma			
Penetrating	2	2	1
Open head	1	1	1
Closed head	6	6	3
Residual	4	4	2
Toxic			
Alcoholic CBS	11	10	9
Carbon monoxide	1	1	1
Vascular			
Malformation (operated)	2	2	1
Cerebral vascular accident	13	13	8
Arteriosclerosis	6	6	4
Tumor			
Unoperated	2	1	2
Post operative	1	1	1
Degenerative process			
Cerebral atrophy	4	4	2
Huntington's chorea	2	2	2
Multiple sclerosis	6	6	2
Myotonia atrophica	1	1	0
Diseases (neurological)			
Abscess (operated)	1	1	1
Encephalitis	2	2	0
Meningitis	1	1	0
Congenital	9	9	9
Undetermined etiology	5	5	2
Control subjects			
Neurosis	6	6	5
Convulsive disorder	2	2	2
Optic nerve atrophy	1	1	1
Peripheral neuritis	1	1	1
Spinal conditions	9	9	7
Unspecified (observation)	7	7	6
Totals	106	104	73
Total controls	26	26	22

These six categories (controls excluded) contained 51 cases or 64% of the brain damaged cases in the total pool. The rest of the cases were spread over the remaining 14 categories. Cerebral vascular accident was the brain damaged category with the largest number of cases but it only contained 13 cases. Thus it was evident that no single diagnostic category dominated the subject pool. Seventeen of the brain damaged cases had multiple diagnoses, but not of the types that would have eliminated them from the pool.

The control group also contained patients in several different diagnostic categories. Of the 26 cases, seven had various forms of neurosis, while the remainder had neurological conditions that did not affect the cerebral cortex, such as spinal cord conditions. The optic atrophy case did not have cortical damage associated with this condition, and the spinal cord cases had low cord lesions such that arm movements were not affected. The cases classified as "unspecified" consisted mainly of patients who were in the hospital for observation and evaluation. They did not have formal diagnoses at the time they were tested, but they had received neurological examinations that were negative for the brain.

TESTING PROCEDURE

This study utilized cases which had been given the Halstead Neuropsychological Battery as adapted by G. Goldstein and P. Rennick. The cases referred to this laboratory were tested as available and the results were filed to be used in many different studies of which this was one. Subjects were tested and the results scored individually by trained testers according to standard procedures (Reitan, 1966). The neuropsychologist examined the scored test results, rated the aphasia examination, the spatial relations and the perceptual disorders tests and then averaged the results of the 12 tests that constitute the "index" tests. These final results were placed on two types of summary sheets. From these final results the psychologist wrote the neuropsychological report on an inferential basis. An example of this procedure is given in Chapter 4. This report was written without knowledge of the subject's neurological results, his history or even seeing the subject. Consequently the only available information given to the neuropsychologist was the test scores plus the patient's age, occupation and education.

All of the test results along with the neuropsychologist's report, the neurologist's report and patient's history were filed together. In this research study the Keys utilized most but not all of the tests that make up the standard neuropsychological battery.

TREATMENT OF DATA

The procedures used in placing the cases into the various Key categories has been presented in Chapter 6. Briefly, this involved inspection and classification of the neurological and neuropsychological reports, and "running" of the Key. In order to reduce possible bias effects, the Key running was accomplished by a clerk who had no formal knowledge of neurology or psychology, and who did not know the aims of the study.[1] He had the tasks of converting the raw test scores to ratings, and of applying the Key to each case according to the instructions presented in Chapter 4.

The data obtained consisted of the numbers of subjects placed into the various categories in each of the two major keys, by each of the three methods. The aim of the data analysis was to evaluate extent of agreement among methods. The major objective was to ascertain the extent of agreement between the Key and the neurological report, but analyses were also made in which the Key was compared with the neuropsychological report, and in which the neuropsychological report was compared with the neurological report. These comparisons may be accomplished by generating three multiple contingency tables. One of them compares the Key with the neurological report, the second, the neuropsychological report with the neurological report, and the third, the Key with the neuropsychological report. Two sets of these multiple contingency tables were constructed; one for the Localization Key and one for the Process Key.

Each of the tables contains cells for each of the four possible classifications, for example, not brain damaged, left hemisphere, right hemisphere, and diffuse. Classifications assigned by one method are placed across the horizontal axis, and classifications assigned by a second method are placed across the vertical axis. Agreements line up along one of the diagonals. Disagreements would appear in those cells that do not line up on the chosen diagonal.

The purpose of the statistical analysis of these tables was to determine whether or not more agreement was obtained than would be expected on the basis of random assignment to cells. Although, theoretically, one agreement out of four would occur on a chance basis, the existence of obvious population biases led the authors to compute their expected frequencies on the basis of the marginal totals of the contingency tables. A statistic was needed to test for the significance of degree of agreement for nominal data. Chi-square techniques are not the methods of choice since chi-square evaluates degree of association, which is not necessarily the same thing as degree of agreement. Exceedingly high chi-square values can

[1] Appreciation is expressed to James K. Majors for his contribution to this research.

be obtained with close to complete disagreement. Cohen's Kappa coefficient (Cohen, 1960) was chosen as the most appropriate statistic. Kappa is a coefficient of agreement for nominal scales. Kappa may range from +1 (perfect agreement) to −1 (perfect disagreement). Kappa is computed by subtracting the proportion of obtained agreements from the proportion of agreements that would be expected by chance, and dividing through by 1 minus the proportion of agreements that would be expected by chance. The significance of Kappa may be tested by dividing it by its standard error and referring the resulting critical ratio to a standard normal distribution table.

Agreement was always determined in a way that involved consideration of the entire pool of subjects for the Key being evaluated. If one method, for example, the neuropsychological report, classified a subject into the same category as another method, then an agreement was obtained. It may be pointed out that this method may, in some situations, produce artifactual results, since the amount of agreement may be inflated or reduced by varying the number of categories, or by constructing categories such that good or poor agreement may be obtained as desired. However, in the case of the present study the categories used were based on dimensions traditionally found in the neurological and neuropsychological literature.

Two kinds of validity were evaluated in this study. The first kind involved a comparison of the Key with neurological examinational findings. For purposes of the present study, the neurological examination is the ultimate criterion. The second validation procedure concerned the accuracy with which the Key replicated the conclusions reached by the neuropsychologist. The authors also wished to ascertain whether one of the two methods was more accurate in predicting neurological findings than the other. This step was accomplished by comparing conclusions found in the neuropsychological reports with neurological findings. In this way a determination could be made of whether or not there was a difference between the Key and the inferential method in regard to level of accuracy in predicting to neurological criteria. Such a difference can be determined by simple inspection of the percentages of correct prediction made by each of the methods. However, chi-square tests were also used in order to determine whether observed differences were statistically significant.

Analyses were also performed for evaluating total agreement (i.e., degree of consistency among the three methods; the Key, the neuropsychological inferential technique and the neurological examination). A chi-square method was employed here since the Kappa coefficient did not appear to be usable in this instance. Direction of any association found was assessed by inspection and by an evaluation of each cell's contribution to the overall chi-square value obtained.

Finally, the validity of each of the individual Key categories was evaluated. This analysis indicated whether or not, for example, the left hemisphere category contains more or less agreements than the diffuse category. A method of mutual inclusion and exclusion comparisons was used here (i.e., a count is made of the number of times two of the methods agreed to assign or not assign a case into a particular category). Such comparisons were made for the Key versus the neurological examination, the Key versus the neuropsychological report and the neuropsychological report vs. the neurological examination. The results of this analysis were also evaluated with chi-square tests. The purpose of this validation procedure was that of determining whether or not there were relatively "strong" and "weak" categories in terms of degree of agreement.

CHAPTER 8

Results

Results are presented in terms of degree of agreement among the three diagnostic methods (i.e., the Key, the neuropsychological report and the neurological examination). The first aspect of the study to be taken up is a consideration of extent of agreement between (a) the Key and the neurological examination, and (b) the neuropsychological report and the neurological examination. The second area of investigation to be considered concerns the extent of agreement between the Key and the neuropsychological report. The validity of each of the individual categories of diagnostic classifications made by the Key and the neuropsychological report were ascertained through determination of the extent of agreement with neurological examinational findings. A determination of the extent of agreement between the Key and the neuropsychological report for the individual categories is also presented. All of these evaluations are presented for the Localization and Process Keys separately.

A brief summary of the major results is reported first, after which more detailed information is provided. Agreement was reached among all three diagnostic methods at highly statistically significant levels. For the Localization Key percentages of agreement were as follows: Key versus neurological examination, 55.8%; neuropsychological report versus neurological examination, 67.3%; Key versus neuropsychological report, 64.4%. For the Process Key percentages of agreement were as follows: Key versus neurological examination, 74.0%; neuropsychological report versus neurological examination, 72.6%; Key versus neuropsychological report, 75.3%. It may be pointed out that these percentages refer to complete agreement, including presence or absence of brain damage and localization or process. Percentages of agreement for presence or absence of brain damage alone were substantially higher. The analysis of individual categories of the Localization Key yielded percentages of agreement between the Key and the neurological examination ranging from 62.5 to 88.5%. For the comparison between the neuropsychological report and the neurological examination level of agreement ranged between 73.1 and 89.4%. For the comparison between the Key and the neuropsychological report the range extended from 72.1 to 87.5%. In all of these comparisons higher levels of agreement were found for the right and left hemisphere categories than for the diffuse category. The corresponding results for the Process Key are as follows: Agreement between the Key and the neurological examination ranged from 76.7 to 93.2%. For the comparison between the neuropsychological report and the neurological examination the range of agreement was from 78.1 to 91.8%. For the comparison between the Key and the neuropsychological report the range was from 87.7 to 93.2%. Here, higher levels of agreement were found for the acute and congenital categories than for the static category. It may be pointed out that these percentages are based on mutual inclusions and exclusions and should not be interpreted as reflecting complete agreement. They only reflect agreement as to whether a case should or should not be included in a particular category.

LOCALIZATION KEY RESULTS

Comparison of Key and Neurological Examinational Findings

The pattern of agreements and disagreements between the Key and the neurological findings for each of the four categories used in the Localization Key is presented in Table 6. The agreements will be found along the diagonal running from the lower left to the upper right corner of the table. Overall, 58 of the 104 *S*s received a Key diagnosis that agreed with the neurological report (55.8% agreement). With regard to presence or absence of brain damage, there were only seven cases (6.7%) in which the Key predicted brain damage that was not confirmed by neurological examination, and five cases (4.8%) in which the Key did not detect brain damage but the neurological examination did. The other disagreements involved the question of localization.

Table 6. Localization Study; Comparison of Key and Neurological Examination Results for Four Categories of Brain Damage

	Neurological				
Key	Not Brain Damaged	Right	Diffuse	Left	Totals
Left	0	1	11	13	25
Diffuse	6	4	19	5	34
Right	1	9	11	2	23
Not brain damaged	17	2	2	1	22
Totals	24	16	43	21	104

Statistical analysis of the data presented in Table 6 was accomplished by using the Kappa coefficient method, in which chance was a function of the marginal distributions. This estimate will set the probability of agreement by chance higher than would an assumption that the probability of agreement is 1 in 4. The obtained Kappa coefficient was .40 (z = 7.33), a value that is significant beyond the .001 level of confidence. It would appear that there is a high degree of agreement between the Key and neurological examination in terms of localization of brain damage. Most of the disagreements occurred in those cases in which the Key predicted a lateralized lesion, while the neurological finding was that the patient had a diffuse lesion. One possible source for this disagreement is that the neuropsychological battery may be more sensitive than the neurological examination to differences in functioning between the cerebral hemispheres.

Comparison of Neuropsychological Clinical Report and Neurological Examination

In order to determine how well the Key agreed with neurological examinational findings as compared with the clinical interpretations made by the neuropsychologist, the neuropsychological reports were validated against neurological criteria. The pattern of agreements and disagreements between these reports and neurological examinational findings is presented in Table 7. Among the 104 *S*s there was agreement in 70 cases (67.3% agreement). With regard to presence or absence of brain damage, in six cases (5.8%) brain damage was predicted in the neuropsychological report but was not confirmed by neurological examination, whereas in five cases (4.8%) brain damage was detected on neurological examination but was not predicted in the neuropsychological report. The remainder of the disagreements had to do with the question of localization. Again the major source of disagreement was found in those cases in which the neuropsychological report stated that the patient had a lateralized lesion, whereas the neurological findings indicated a diffuse lesion.

Statistical analysis of the data presented in Table 7 was again accomplished through employment of the Kappa coefficient. The obtained Kappa was .55 (z = 10.17), a value significant beyond the .001 level. Thus the clinical interpretation method agrees with neurological findings in terms of localization at a level far exceeding chance. Since correct agreement overall was obtained in 56% of the cases using the Key and 67% of the cases using clinical interpretation, the clinical interpretation method is a bit more accurate. Statistically, however, the two methods are not significantly different from each other in regard to level of agreement. The frequencies of correct and incorrect predictions were placed into a fourfold contingency table and the chi-square value was computed. A chi-square of 2.92

Table 7. Localization Study; Comparison of the Neuropsychological Assessment Results with the Neurological Examination Results for Four Categories of Brain Damage

	Neurological				
Neuropsychological	Not Brain Damaged	Right	Diffuse	Left	Totals
Left	2	1	7	15	25
Diffuse	3	4	26	4	37
Right	1	11	7	0	19
Not brain damaged	18	0	3	2	23
Totals	24	16	43	21	104

was obtained, which is not significant at the .05 level. It therefore cannot be concluded that either method is superior to the other in terms of accuracy of prediction of neurological criteria.

In view of the above findings it would be reasonable to conclude that the clinician who wishes to limit his report to what can be expressed by the Key can do so, knowing that he will probably make many more correct predictions than would be expected by chance. In view of the general shortage of clinical psychologists and the far greater shortage of clinicians trained in neuropsychology the authors feel that the Key may be of use in a number of clinical applications at the present time. Hopefully, future refinements of the Key will augment its usefulness.

Comparison of Key and Neuropsychological Clinical Report

This comparison does not involve validation against neurological criteria, but rather focuses on how well the Key and the neuropsychologist's clinical interpretation agree with each other. In those situations, mentioned above, in which a neuropsychologist is not available, there may be a desire

Table 8. Localization Study; Comparison of Key and Neuropsychological Test Results for Four Categories of Brain Damage

	Neuropsychological				
Key	Not Brain Damaged	Right	Diffuse	Left	Totals
Left	2	1	4	18	25
Diffuse	5	3	21	5	34
Right	0	12	11	0	23
Not brain damaged	16	3	1	2	22
Totals	23	19	37	25	104

to substitute the Key for clinical interpretation. It would then be of value to know how well the Key approximates the neuropsychologist's assessment in regard to the diagnostic categories used here. This comparison was made using the same methods employed above. The agreement and disagreement pattern is presented in Table 8. In 67 of the 104 cases complete agreement was obtained (64.4%). With regard to presence or absence of brain damage, seven (6.7%) were classified as brain damaged by the Key and not brain damaged by the neuropsychological report; six cases (5.8%) were classified as brain damaged by the neuropsychological report and not brain damaged by the Key. The remaining disagreements had to do with the question of localization.

Inspection of Table 8 reveals that there are 11 cases in which the Key predicts a right-hemisphere lesion, whereas the neuropsychological report predicts a diffuse lesion. This discrepancy appears to represent the major source of disagreement. Either the Key overdiagnoses right-hemisphere dysfunction or the neuropsychological report underdiagnoses it. This finding is consistent with the present lack of knowledge concerning the psychological functions of the right cerebral hemisphere as compared with far more extensive information about the left hemisphere.

Again, a Kappa coefficient was computed in order to determine the level of statistical significance for overall agreement. Kappa was found to be equal to .51 ($z = 9.69$), a value significant beyond the .001 level. It can be concluded that there is a high degree of agreement between predictions made on a clinical interpretation basis by the neuropsychologist and those made by the Key.

Total Agreement

So far it has been shown that the Key and the neuropsychological report can predict neurological findings with a high degree of accuracy, and that there is a high level of agreement between the Key and the neuropsychological report. It has also been shown that while the method of clinical interpretation is somewhat more accurate than the Key in predicting the neurological diagnosis, the difference in frequencies of correct classifications is not statistically significant. In this section two analyses will be presented, both of which have the aim of ascertaining the extent of agreement among the three methods, that is, the neurological examination, the neuropsychological clinical interpretation and the Key. First, a chi-square test was employed to determine whether or not there was a statistically significant degree of association among the three methods. The contingency table for this measure is presented in Table 9. It was found that a three-way agreement occurred in 50 of 104 cases. Chi-square was found to be equal to 245.52, a value significant beyond the .001 level. The contingency coeffi-

Table 9. Localization Study; Total Agreement Between the Results of the Key, the Neuropsychological Reports and the Neurological Examination; Table of Observed and Expected Frequencies

	Three Agree	Two Agree	None Agree
Expected frequencies	7.98	59.52	36.50
Obtained frequencies	50.0	45.0	9.0
Contribution to overall χ^2	221.26	3.54	20.139

cient was equal to .83, a value also significant beyond the .001 level. These results indicate that there was a very high level of agreement among the Key, the neuropsychological report and the neurological examinational findings.

Another way of examining relationships among the three methods involves a comparison of the Key and the neuropsychological report with respect to frequency of agreement with neurological findings. That is, one can count the number of times the Key and the neuropsychological report both agree with the neurological findings, the number of times one agrees and the other disagrees, and the number of times that both the Key and the neuropsychological report disagree with the neurological examinational findings. The obtained frequencies in each of these categories are presented in Table 10. It will be noted that in 50 of the 104 cases the Key and the neuropsychological report agreed in correctly predicting the neurological findings. The resulting chi-square is equal to 244.09, a value significant beyond the .001 level of confidence. Again, it has been demonstrated that there is a highly significant level of agreement among the three methods.

Analysis of Individual Categories

Although the Localization Key appears to be valid as a whole, it was felt that the relative accuracy of the individual categories (i.e., not brain

Table 10. Localization Study; Prediction of the Neurological Examination Results by the Key and the Neuropsychological Reports in Frequencies of Correct (+) and Incorrect (−) Predictions

		Neuropsychological −	Neuropsychological +
Key	+	E = 19.74 O = 8.00	E = 7.98 O = 50.00
	−	E = 55.69 O = 26.00	E = 20.59 O = 20.00

Table 11. Localization Study; Percent of Correct Predictions of the Neurological Examination Report by the Key for Four Individual Localization Categories

Category	No. of Agreements	Disagreements: No. of False Negatives	Disagreements: No. of False Positives	Percent of Agreements	χ^2
Left	84	12	8	80.76	20.65
Diffuse	65	15	24	62.50	4.40
Right	83	14	7	79.80	12.78
Not brain damaged	92	5	7	88.46	46.13

damaged, diffuse, right hemisphere, and left hemisphere) should also be examined. By doing so the areas of relative strength and weakness of the Key can be identified and appropriate corrections made in future versions.

Results of the evaluation of the individual categories are presented in Tables 11, 12 and 13 in terms of percentages and frequencies of agreeing and disagreeing upon the classifications, comparing the Key and the neurological examinational findings, the neuropsychological report and the neurological examinational findings, and the Key and the neuropsychological report. The data presented in Tables 11–13 were computed in the following way. Agreements were defined as mutual inclusions and exclusions; that is, if the two methods being compared agreed as to a particular classification, or if they agreed that the case in question did not fit that classification, then the case was counted as an agreement. Thus in each comparison the base for computing percentages was always the entire sample of 104 *S*s. It will be noted that this definition of agreement differs from that used in the overall comparisons. In those analyses, only mutual inclusion in a particular category was considered to be an agreement. In the analysis of individual categories the method of defining agreement used

Table 12. Localization Study; Percent of Correct Predictions of the Neurological Examination Report by the Neuropsychological Report for Four Individual Localization Categories

Category	No. of Agreements	Disagreements: No. of False Negatives	Disagreements: No. of False Positives	Percent of Agreements	χ^2
Left	88	10	6	84.62	32.34
Diffuse	78	11	17	73.08	19.81
Right	91	8	5	87.50	32.32
Not brain damaged	91	5	6	89.42	50.63

in the overall comparisons is obviously not appropriate, since here the objective is to determine the degree of agreement in the categories taken one at a time. An example may clarify this matter. Let us take the case of the comparison between the Key and the neurological examination with regard to the not brain damaged category. Inspection of Table 11 will reveal that there were 92 agreements. This means that in 92 of the 104 cases, the Key and the neurological examination agreed with regard to presence or absence of brain damage. It does not imply perfect agreement in those 92 cases. In several of them classified as brain damaged, there was disagreement as to whether the lesion was in the right hemisphere, the left hemisphere or diffuse. These disagreements, however, are irrelevant to assessment of accuracy in prediction of the not brain damaged category taken individually. Looking at the various categories individually, it appears that the ability of the Key to discriminate between brain damaged and nonbrain damaged cases is quite adequate. It agreed with the neurological di-

Table 13. Localization Study; Percent of Correct Predictions of the Neuropsychological Report by the Key for Four Individual Localization Categories

		Disagreements			
Category	**No. of Agreements**	**No. of False Negatives**	**No. of False Positives**	**Percent of Agreements**	χ^2
Left	**90**	**7**	**7**	**86.53**	**41.46**
Diffuse	**75**	**13**	**16**	**72.11**	**15.10**
Right	**86**	**11**	**7**	**82.69**	**22.75**
Not brain damaged	**91**	**6**	**7**	**87.50**	**41.44**

agnosis in 88.6% of the cases. This level of accuracy approximates the level achieved with the use of the Halstead impairment index (Halstead, 1947; Wheeler and Reitan, 1963). It is also approximately equivalent to the cross-validation results of a linear discriminant function analysis performed by Wheeler and Reitan (1963). In evaluating these results it should be borne in mind that the entire control group had been referred for neuropsychological testing because of suspected brain damage. Thus, even though the neurological examination was negative, many of these cases may have had residual cerebral dysfunction, thereby reducing their value as a sample of nonbrain damaged *S*s.

The ability of the Key to select the neurologically diagnosed nonbrain damaged cases was about the same as that of the neuropsychological clinical method, as indicated in Table 10. The possibility has already been suggested that the neuropsychological examination may be more sensitive to cortical dysfunction than the neurological examination. A consequence of this situation is that in the case of the present control group, there may be some cases with borderline conditions that might be categorized as brain damaged or not, almost as a matter of chance. Clearly, such a condition would tend to reduce the accuracy of the Key as we have been measuring it. Despite this handicap there was a high degree of agreement between neurological and neuropsychological methods with regard to the presence or absence of brain damage.

Further inspection of Table 11 reveals that the Key is at its weakest in the diffuse category. It only agrees with neurological findings 62.50% of the time. As has been pointed out in the section on the comparison of the Key with neurological findings (see Table 6), a major source of error is the tendency of the Key to lateralize cases that the neurologists call diffuse. The possibility that the Key is more sensitive to lateralized deficit than the neurological examination was suggested, but the nature of lateralized deficit in a number of neurological diseases is also a crucial consideration. Many disease entities may give rise to both lateralized and diffuse effects in the same patient. There may be damage to both cerebral hemispheres, but one is more involved than the other. This picture is typical, for example, in cerebral vascular accidents. Often the neuropsychological report stated that the patient had both lateralized and diffuse damage, but for purposes of the present study the neuropsychologist had to re-examine these cases and force them into either the diffuse or the lateralized category. In many cases such a decision was rather arbitrary, and this situation was reflected in the relatively low percentage of agreement with neurological findings in regard to the diffuse category.

The results for the lateralized categories are substantially more satisfactory. Amount of agreement here ranges from 79.8 to 80.8%. The Key's ability to identify lateralized cases was similar to that of the neuropsychological report. Inspection of Table 8 will also reveal that in only one case was there a disagreement between the Key and the neuropsychological report in regard to the side of the lesion in those cases in which lateralization was predicted by both methods. Only three disagreements of this type were found in the comparison of the Key with neurological findings (see Table 6), and only one was found in the case of the predictions made by the neuropsychological report (see Table 7).

A major source of disagreement in the Key appeared to be its tendency to lateralize to the right cerebral hemisphere in many cases that were diagnosed as diffuse by the neurologists. This tendency was also present for the left hemisphere, but not to so great an extent. The Key also tended to lateralize more cases than did the neuropsychological examination. If one wishes to gain higher agreement with neurological findings, some selective readjustment of cutting points may be made. However, the lateralizing information provided by the Key, even in cases in which it does not agree with neurological diagnosis, may be of some significance in understanding the patient's behavior. Thus the clinician may desire that the Key retain its present sensitivity to lateralized deficit if the postulation of such deficit is supported by observation of the patient's behavior.

PROCESS KEY RESULTS

There is a great deal of evidence demonstrating that the kinds of psychological dysfunction seen are related to the localization of the brain lesion. Consequently, one would expect that a Key could be built which categorized brain damage according to location. The question arises as to whether a Key could be constructed to categorize other aspects of brain damage; that is, can the type of brain damage be predicted as well as the location. This matter is of particular significance since Reitan has pointed out that there is an interaction between location and type of lesion in determining the behavioral outcome. A lesion in a particular locus can produce various behavioral consequences depending on the kind of lesion it is; for example, vascular lesions of the left cerebral hemisphere do not produce the same sorts of functional changes as do lesions to the same hemisphere produced by demyelinating disease. What will be called a Process Key was therefore developed in order to deal with this problem. The validation procedure for this Key was the same as that just presented for the Localization Key.

Comparison of Key and Neurological Results

The Process Key utilizes four categories: (a) no brain damage or control *S*s, (b) acute brain damage, (c) static brain damage, (d) congenital brain damage. Definitions of these categories may be found on page 88. The

Table 14. Process Study; Comparison of Key and Neurological Examination Results for Four Process Categories of Brain Damage

	Neurological				
Key	**Not Brain Damaged**	**Acute**	**Static**	**Congenital**	**Totals**
Congenital	0	1	5	6	12
Static	6	1	26	2	35
Acute	0	6	2	1	9
Not brain damaged	16	0	1	0	17
Totals	22	8	34	9	73

Table 15. Process Study; Comparison of the Neuropsychological Assessment Results with the Neurological Examination Results for Four Categories of Brain Damage

	Neurological				
Neuropsychological	**Not Brain Damaged**	**Acute**	**Static**	**Congenital**	**Totals**
Congenital	2	0	5	6	13
Static	3	2	24	1	30
Acute	0	6	2	2	10
Not brain damaged	17	0	3	0	20
Totals	22	8	34	9	73

tabulation of agreements and disagreements between the Key and the neurological findings are presented in Table 14. Again, the agreements will be found along the diagonal going from the lower left to the upper right corner of the table. Complete agreement was obtained in 54 (74.0%) of the cases. With regard to presence or absence of brain damage, in six cases (8.2%) the Key predicted brain damage that was not confirmed by neurological examination. In one case (1.4%) brain damage was diagnosed by neurological examination but was not identified by the Key. The remaining disagreements had to do with identification of the process. Most of them were cases in which the Key predicted a congenital process while the neurological diagnosis was static brain damage.

Statistical analysis again utilized the Kappa coefficient. The obtained Kappa was .61 (z = 7.96), a value significant beyond the .001 level. Thus the Key can predict process neurological diagnosis at a level far exceeding chance.

Comparison of Neuropsychological Clinical Prediction with Neurological Results

The pattern of agreements and disagreements between the neuropsychological clinical predictions of process and the neurological examinational results is presented in Table 15. Among the 73 *S*s there were 53 complete agreements (72.6%). With regard to presence or absence of brain damage, there were five cases (6.8%) for which the neuropsychologist predicted brain damage not confirmed by neurological examination, and three cases (4.1%) in which brain damage was found on neurological examination but was not detected by the neuropsychologist. The remaining disagreements had to do with the specific processes. Again, the major source of disagreement here involved the tendency for the neuropsychologist to predict congenital brain damage in several cases in which static brain damage was diagnosed by the neurologists. The obtained Kappa coefficient was found to be equal to .60 (z = 7.82), a value significant beyond the .001 level. Thus the neuropsychologist can predict the neurological process diagnosis at a level that far exceeds chance.

In regard to the question of process the Key did a bit better than the neuropsychologist. It obtained complete agreement in 54 (74.0%) of the 73 cases, whereas the clinical method obtained complete agreement in 53 of the cases (72.6%). In order to determine whether these differences are statistically significant, the frequencies of agreements and disagreements for both methods were placed into a fourfold contingency table and a chi-square test was performed. Chi-square was found to be equal to .03, a value not statistically significant at the .05 level. As was the case for the Localization Key, neither method did better than the other in terms of complete agreement with neurological diagnosis.

COMPARISON OF THE KEY AND THE NEUROPSYCHOLOGICAL CLINICAL PREDICTION METHODS

The pattern of agreements and disagreements between the Process Key and the neuropsychologist's predictions is presented in Table 16. Of the 73 *S*s, complete agreement was obtained for 55 of the cases (75.3%). With regard to presence or absence of brain damage, there were six cases (8.2%) in which brain damage was predicted by the Key but not by the neuropsychologist, and three cases (4.1%) in which the neuropsychologist predicted brain damage but the Key did not. The remaining disagreements had to do with the specific process involved, but there does not appear to be a predominant source of disagreement, except perhaps for some slight tendency to differ as to whether or not the *S* has an acute or static lesion. The Kappa coefficient obtained was equal to .64 (z = 8.36), a value significant beyond the .001 level. It would appear that the degree of agreement be-

Table 16. Process Study; Comparison of Key and Neuropsychological Assessment Results for Four Process Categories of Brain Damage

	Neuropsychological				
Key	**Not Brain Damaged**	**Acute**	**Static**	**Congenital**	**Totals**
Congenital	0	1	1	10	12
Static	6	3	25	1	35
Acute	0	6	3	0	9
Not brain damaged	14	0	1	2	17
Totals	20	10	30	13	73

Table 17. Process Study: Total Agreement Between the Results of the Key, the Neuropsychological Reports and the Neurological Examination; Table of Observed and Expected Frequencies

	Three Agree	Two Agree	None Agree
Expected frequencies	8.50	43.50	21.00
Obtained frequencies	46.0	24.0	3.0
Contribution to overall χ^2	165.44	8.74	15.43

tween the Key and the neuropsychologist is significantly greater than would be expected on the basis of chance.

Total Agreement

The same methods of analysis used to ascertain the extent of agreement among the three methods for the Localization Key were applied to the Process Key. A chi-square test was employed to determine whether or not there was a statistically significant degree of association among the three methods. The contingency table for this measure is presented in Table 17. Since the marginal probabilities for process are different from those obtained in the localization study, the probabilities of chance agreement also change. The obtained chi-square was found to be equal to 189.61, a value significant beyond the .001 level. The contingency coefficient is .85, which is also statistically significant beyond the .001 level. These results indicate that the extent of interagreement among the three methods is far greater than what would be expected on the basis of chance.

A comparison of the Key and the neuropsychological report with respect to frequency of agreement with neurological findings was also made. The pertinent obtained and expected frequencies are presented in Table 18. A chi-square value of 187.68 was obtained, which is significant beyond the .001 level. The contingency coefficient is .85, which is also sig-

Table 18. Process Study; Prediction of the Neurological Examination Results by the Key and the Neuropsychological Reports in Frequencies of Correct (+) and Incorrect (−) Predictions

		Neuropsychological −	Neuropsychological +
Key	+	E = 15.39 O = 8.00	E = 8.50 O = 46.00
Key	−	E = 34.91 O = 12.00	E = 14.20 O = 7.00

nificant beyond the .001 level. The reader is reminded that the expected frequencies used for these analyses were obtained from the marginal totals of the contingency tables. Results of both of these analyses reveal that there is a high degree of interagreement among the three methods with regard to diagnosis of process.

Analysis of Individual Categories

Frequencies and percentages of agreement among the various methods for each of the Process Key categories are presented in Tables 19–21. They were computed in the same manner as described in the corresponding section for the Localization Key. Inspection of these tables reveal a generally high level of agreement among all three methods. A comparison of Tables 19–21 with Tables 11–13 indicates that there is a tendency toward higher levels of interagreement with the Process Key than with the Localization Key. Perhaps one reason for this is that the assignment of *S*s

Table 19. Process Study; Percent of Correct Predictions of the Neurological Examination Report by the Key for Four Individual Process Categories

Category	No. of Agreements	Disagreements: No. of False Negatives	Disagreements: No. of False Positives	Percent of Agreements	χ^2
Congenital	64	6	3	87.67	18.84
Static	56	9	8	76.71	20.75
Acute	68	3	2	93.15	32.51
Not brain damaged	66	1	6	90.41	43.12

to localization categories was somewhat more arbitrary than was the case with the process categories, since they contained cases in the right and left hemisphere groups that had both lateralized and diffuse symptoms. As was mentioned above, the neuropsychologist had to place such cases into either the diffuse or one of the lateralized categories in accordance with his subjective judgments of degree of lateralized dysfunction. It would appear that the process categories are somewhat more objective since they are defined in terms of disease entity and time since acquisition of the lesion. In this regard it is interesting to note that the static category, which is the least well defined one, is also the one in which the poorest levels of agreement were generally obtained.

Other reasons for the slight superiority of the Process Key over the Localization Key were, first, that some of the more difficult, borderline cases were eliminated from consideration in the analysis of the Process Key re-

Table 20. Process Study; Percent of Correct Predictions of the Neurological Examination Report by the Neuropsychological Report for Four Individual Process Categories

Category	No. of Agreements	Disagreements: No. of False Negatives	Disagreements: No. of False Positives	Percent of Agreements	χ^2
Congenital	63	7	3	86.30	16.78
Static	57	6	10	78.08	22.88
Acute	67	4	2	91.78	28.43
Not brain damaged	65	3	5	89.04	39.35

sults. These were cases in which process was not specified by the neuropsychologist. Four borderline control cases that were included in the Localization Key pool were not included in the Process Key pool for this reason. In these cases the neuropsychological report had stated that they were brain damaged but failed to state the process involved. Second, the Process Key as a whole predicted slightly better than the Localization Key. This difference is also probably attributable to the fact that the Process Key categories were more well defined and the cases used were more clear cut.

Inspection of Tables 19, 20, and 21 indicates that generally the lowest degree of agreement was found for the static category. To a certain extent this category was residual in nature whereas the acute and congenital categories were better defined from the point of view of the Key as well as that of the neurological examination. The acute category was limited to the immediate effects of head trauma, CVAs and fast growing tumors. The congenital category was also fairly specific, being limited to cases of brain lesions occurring during the perinatal period. Everything else was placed into the static category. Hopefully further elaboration of the Process Key will differentiate among the groups placed into the static category. In the

Table 21. Process Study; Percent of Correct Predictions of the Neuropsychological Report by the Key for Four Individual Process Categories

Category	No. of Agreements	Disagreements: No. of False Negatives	Disagreements: No. of False Positives	Percent of Agreements	χ^2
Congenital	68	2	3	93.15	42.05
Static	58	10	5	79.45	25.57
Acute	66	3	4	90.41	24.43
Not brain damaged	64	3	6	87.67	33.62

present study various diagnostic groups (e.g., old head traumas and residual CVAs) were lumped together, which lowered the percent of agreement.

In the case of the congenital category the level of agreement between the Key and the neuropsychological report was slightly higher than between the Key and the neurological examination, and between the neuropsychological report and the neurological examination. Examination of Tables 14 and 15 reveals that for both the Key and the neuropsychological report there were 5 cases in which a predicted congenital lesion was called static by the neurologists. This lack of agreement may be partially attributable to differences among neurologists with regard to the diagnosis of congenital lesions. Differences of opinion with regard to, for example, time after birth allowed in diagnosing the lesion as congenital may have produced some variability in classification of cases. Since congenital lesions are usually static, in the absence of an adequate history many neurologists may not wish to postulate the existence of a congenital lesion as opposed to static brain damage acquired later in life. However, the Process Key was quite successful in replicating the inference pattern used by the neuropsychologist in predicting congenital brain damage.

CHAPTER 9

General Discussion

VALIDITY OF THE KEYING PROCEDURE

The principal results of this research indicate that the keying procedure used in this study proved to be valid. This validity was demonstrated for both the Localization and Process Keys. Agreement was obtained with both the neurological results and the neuropsychological examination results in regard to the categories of brain damage used beyond the .001 level of significance. These categories were major ones for the localization of brain damage (right hemisphere, left hemisphere, and diffuse) and for various kinds of brain damage (acute, static, and congenital).

These Keys need cross validation studies which could not be done at this laboratory since the original study had exhausted the available subject pool. Some drop in the levels of agreement would probably occur initially, though with further research on these Keys the final agreement should be at least as high as that found in the present study. One difficulty that may arise in a cross validation study is that the present Keys have been designed to fit the neuropsychological program at one laboratory quite closely and some revision may need to be made, especially in the cutting points, to fit them to other laboratories. The population of patients will vary somewhat from setting to setting according to the type of patients admitted to the neurological service and to the procedures for selecting neuropsychological subjects. Also, at times, a neuropsychologist who is working closely with a particular group of neurologists may develop inferential norms that fit the predilections of those neurologists at least for the standard physical neurological examination. In any case the scaling of the various measures and revision of the cutting points needs to be re-established on a more sound statistical basis than they were in this study.

As a consequence of the validation of these particular Keys it has been demonstrated that valid Keys can be built to diagnose types of brain damage. So far Keys related to only part of the possible classes in only two dimensions of brain damage, localization and process, have been constructed. Since neuropsychologists can isolate other categories of brain damage within these dimensions and also frequently separate out specific disease processes, which is another dimension, there is no theoretical reason why Keys cannot be expanded far beyond the limits of those used in this study. Certainly Biological Keys are almost infinitely extendable. One book in that field may literally key thousands of species.

Comparison with the Inferential Process

Although secondary to the primary concern of this study, the validity of the inferential process or clinical intuition was also supported in regard to analysis of neuropsychological data. The agreement between the neuropsychologist's "blind" report and the neurological report was found to be quite high for both the localization categories (Table 7) and the process categories (Table 15). In both cases the significance level was beyond .001. This was true for the individual categories in both dimensions of brain damage studies (Tables 12 and 20). The percent correctly predicted ran from 91.8 to 73.1. These results were quite comparable with those found in similar research by Reitan (1964a) and Wheeler and Reitan (1963). The rate of correct prediction of brain damage appears to be higher than clinical inference using the MMPI (Meehl, 1959). This discrepancy may be related to the difference in criteria. The neurological criterion is probably more precise and accurate than the psychiatric diagnosis. As in the case of the MMPI studies (Meehl, 1959; Kleinmuntz, 1963) it is likely that use of an objective method will eventually increase the level of correct prediction or hits above that for the inferential process. The Meehl and Dahlstrom (1960a, 1960b) rules for separating psychotics from neurotics have proved to be especially accurate (Heinrichs, 1964, 1966; Meehl, 1959).

Many of the advantages and disadvantages of the inferential process in relation to objective methods which Meehl (1959) discussed can be found in this study. In regard to open-endedness of clinical judgment or the ability to meet new situations, the neuropsychologist can often take such things as peripheral damage or depression into consideration and "partial out" its effects, something a Key cannot do. In this regard Keys could be made which, to a certain extent, take some unusual situations into consideration; however, a special Key or part of a Key would need to be constructed for each special situation. This procedure is also necessary for what Meehl calls "empty cells," which are unusual or rare instances. Again special Keys could be constructed to include these special cases. Such construction would be a particularly reasonable procedure if computers can be programmed to "run" the keys.

Perhaps the particular advantage of the inferential neuropsychologist's assessment over an established Key is his ability to utilize "theory mediation" (Meehl, 1959); that is, by using a general theory he can determine what the results of certain patterns should be. If he knows that somesthesis is related to contralateral damage, he can state that a man with a right hemianesthesia has damage in his left hemisphere if peripheral damage has been ruled out.

The attempt in Key construction is to build these "theory mediation" concepts into a Key that can be utilized for assessing specific cases. Ultimately a function of the research neuropsychologist may be to produce new theories through his research and then to translate these into keying codes.

The disadvantages of the inferential process were also discussed by Meehl (Meehl, 1959; Meehl & Dahlstrom, 1960a). The ability of psychologists using inferential means of assessing subjects varies a great deal from person to person since generally a great deal of experience is needed to be able to pick out particular patterns. Second, there is a tendency for the clinician's "inferential" cutting points to vary from time to time in a random manner which reduces his accuracy. Finally, the clinician can seldom determine the optimal weights or cutting points as accurately as a well researched objective system.

One area where Meehl initially felt that the clinician had the advantage was in picking out patterns; this he originally thought an objective method could not do. However, he reversed this opinion since his system of rules, which is essentially a key, could do this better than clinical experts (Meehl, 1959). The result is that within its province a Key, whether applied to brain damage or to the MMPI, can duplicate or even better the inferential process used by experienced clinicians in utilizing patterns.

In addition to the work of Meehl, there have been numerous other investigators interested in the clinical versus statistical prediction controversy. Gough's (1962) review of the literature in this area cites studies that date back as far as 1923. Gough epitomizes the crucial issue as follows: "The defining distinction between clinical and actuarial methods is to be found in the way in which the data, once specified, are combined for use in making the prediction. If the procedures, however complex mathematically, are in principle such that a clerk, or a machine, or anyone else could carry out the necessary operations and that the result would be the same in all instances, then the method is actuarial or statistical in the sense here being discussed. If the combining is done intuitively, if hypotheses and constructs are generated during the course of the analysis, and if the process is mediated by an individual's judgment and reflection, then the method is clinical" (p. 530).

A response to Meehl's defense of actuarial methods was made by Holt (1958) who felt that the issue should not have emerged as an either-or controversy, but rather what should be sought is an optimal combination of actuarial and clinical methods aimed at maximizing accurate prediction. Using data from the Holt and Luborsky (1958) study of prediction of success in psychiatry, Holt showed that predictive validity coefficients increased as the amount of information available to judges increased, regardless of whether this information was clinically or statistically derived. In fact, he found that the extent to which the judges liked the psychiatry trainee candidates, clearly an affective, intuitive reaction, was the best statistically significant predictor of success in a psychiatric career. Holt supported the use of what he termed a "sophisticated clinical" approach, which includes application of both qualitative and objective data. He contrasted this method to "naïve clinical" and "pure acturial" approaches, both of which, he felt, have their weaknesses. It is interesting to note that in the present study an actuarial approach (the Neuropsychological Key) was compared with what can probably be classed as a sophisticated clinical approach (the neuropsychological report), with little difference found between them in terms of accuracy of prediction of neurological criteria. The authors of the present study are tempted to suggest that if similar kinds of results are found in future comparative studies of this type, the actuarial method has the distinct advantage of being a far more economical procedure than the sophisticated clinical approach.

Despite Holt's findings, Meehl (1965) has reported that a review of 50 studies done since the publication of his *Clinical versus Statistical Prediction* (1954) revealed that the superiority of the clinical method could not be demonstrated, with one exception. This exception is to be found in a study by Lindzey (1965) in which he compared objectively analyzed Thematic Apperception Test (TAT) protocols with clinical interpretation of these same protocols with the aim of determining which method did best at discriminating between groups of homosexuals and nonhomosexuals. He found that actuarial methods did nearly as well as clinical judgment with a group of college students, but when the study was replicated with a prison population the clinical judgment method was found to be much superior to the actuarial method. In commenting on this study Meehl (1965) suggests that the results may be attributed, in part, to the difficulties inherent in scoring the TAT and to the fact the objectified TAT signs for homosexuality used by Lindzey were clearly shown to be invalid in a prison population. Conceivably, then, if valid signs were available for this population, the clinical and objective methods might have done equally well.

Relationship to the Neurological Examination

There is one final area in which the Key can be compared to the inferential neurological diagnosis of brain damage. The physical neurological examination is weakest in the area of localizing cortical damage. As the central nervous system is descended the localizing ability of the neurological examination improves. In contrast the neuropsychological examination is primarily an examination for cortical damage. In this study some evidence was found to suggest that it may be more sensitive to lateralizing effects than the physical neurological examination; that is, in almost all cases, when the neurological examination lateralized a defect, the neuropsychological examination agreed, as did the Key. Thus in these cases there was little contradiction between the neurological and the neuropsychological examination, nor with the Key. However, cases which the neurological examination considered to be diffuse were often lateralized by the neuropsychological examination and the Key. Thus it was possible that the neuropsychological examination and the Key were picking up indications of lateralized deficit more frequently than the neurological examination.

Using the neurological examination as the criterion, the Key was not quite as accurate as the neuropsychological examination since it tended to lateralize cases more readily than the inferential method in this study. However, further modification of the Key, particularly in regard to the cutting points, may improve its performance. The "sensitiveness" of a Key can be rather easily increased or decreased by either changing the cutting points or changing the number of positive measures needed to indicate a particular category. The optimal way of validating this greater sensitivity would be to follow up a number of progressive brain damage cases that the Key has lateralized and the neurological examination has not. If statistically significant numbers of these cases are later diagnosed as lateralized as the disease processes progress, or as a result of more precise diagnostic studies being done, the sensitivity of the Key will be validated.

THE KEY AS AN OBJECTIVE METHOD

Although the use of a Key is quite venerable in biology, it is new to psychology. However, the two Keys used in this study do not appear to be the first Keys suggested or constructed in psychology though they may be the first to adopt the biological name of Keys. There now exist several psychological "Keys," such as the Meehl and Dahlstrom rules (1960a, 1960b) and various computer programs (Kleinmuntz, 1963), if the rather narrow concept of a Key which biology has generally accepted (Metcalf, 1954) is liberalized to define a Key as any ordered set of rules designed to classify members of a group into two or more categories.

Logical Versus Statistical Structure of a Key

The distinction to be emphasized here is that between a Key and a statistical classifying procedure. A Key is essentially a qualitative or nominal procedure while statistical procedures are quantitative or "nonnominal." Meehl (1959) apparently makes this same distinction indirectly when he distinguishes linear methods, such as the discriminant function, from nonlinear methods, such as the Meehl-Dahlstrom (1960a) rules, for separating psychotic from neurotic MMPI profiles. These rules are given in *An MMPI Handbook* (Dahlstrom & Welsh, 1960, pp. 469–471. Even a cursory examination is sufficient to demonstrate their similarity to the Keys utilized in this study.

Such a set of rules, which constitute a Key, does not use a mathematical method in the quantitative sense, though each individual rule or criterion may be quantitative, but in a rather logical form. This, of course, was also true of the Keys used in this study. These Keys utilize logic or a logical form to gain their objectivity rather than a quantitative form. The utilization of logic as an objective procedure for classifying or diagnosing entities is discussed by Ledley and Lusted (1959). Their analyses of the "reasoning foundation of medical diagnosis" demonstrate how logic can be utilized to objectify an inferential classification procedure. The two Keys in the present study have attempted to translate the inferential process used by professionals in making a "diagnosis" into an objective logical form. The success of this attempt indicates that such a translation can be made. Meehl and Dahlstrom (1960a) also state that the major source of their rules was clinical inferences. In any case the keying method can be considered a nonmathematical procedure for objectively dealing with psychological phenomena.

Logical Hierarchy

The essence of a Key is the logical structure it contains. The logical structure of a Biological Key is quite simple. It is: "A" or "B" and if "A" then "a" or "b" and if "a" then "(1)" or "(2)" (logically "or" is used here as an exclusive disjunction). The key form orders the logic so as to produce a single unified system out of a mere collection of rules. This system is ordered and the order unifies it. This adds a dimension to the decision-making process that an unordered collection of rules does not have. The primary criticism that could be leveled at the Meehl-Dahlstrom rules (Dahlstrom & Welsh, 1960) is that evidently too little attention was paid to their order.

One advantage of a Key is that it can handle certain kinds of qualitative differences that quantitative methods cannot; for instance, to use a rather obvious example, if one wanted to separate humans, dogs and birds, the first criteria could separate out all creatures with two legs. This would categorize dogs but would leave humans and birds together. A second criterion could use a nominal or nonmathematical difference such as the presence or lack of feathers. This would separate humans from birds. The important point is that a logical system can utilize qualitative aspects of psychological material that cannot be legitimately utilized by quantitative methods.

Comparison with Statistical Methods

One of the methods of objectively classifying the MMPI profiles Meehl (1959) examined was the linear discriminant function. This is a complex statistical means of determining the optimal weighting of indicators so as to produce a single coefficient for differentiating groups (Wheeler, Burke & Reitan, 1963). It is certainly one of the most sophisticated statistical techniques for categorizing psychological data and as such it could be considered to be the most accurate statistical technique available. It sets the statistical standard to which Keys could be compared.

Such an analysis has been used in several studies to assess brain damage (Wheeler, 1963; Wheeler & Reitan, 1963; Wheeler, Burke & Reitan, 1963). In the study with Burke and Reitan (1963), Wheeler applied this method to 31 right, 25 left and 23 diffuse brain damaged subjects along with 61 controls. They used the subtests of the Wechsler-Bellevue Scale, most of the Halstead Battery and the Trail Making Test for their behavioral indices. Neurological examinations constituted their criteria. Here the discriminant function could only handle two categories in any one application. It was able to correctly predict right versus left damage in 92.9% of the cases. The rest of the comparisons were between the controls and the three types of brain damage. The percent of correct predictions was in the nineties in all comparisons. Cross validation, however, lowered the percentages 10–20 points (Wheeler & Reitan, 1963). The major study in this cross validation gives these percentages of correct predictions: Control versus all types of brain damage 80%; controls versus diffuse damage 80%; controls versus left-sided damage 80%; controls versus right-sided damage 80%; right versus left 70%; left versus diffuse 70%; and right versus diffuse 65%. The Halstead impairment index was found to be as good as the discriminant function. Thus the cross validation study concludes that ". . . the discriminant function can be expected to produce 75 to 80% CP (correct predictions) in distinguishing between control patients and patients having any one of several categories of cerebral damage. . . . for diffuse or bilateral damage vs. left damage choices of % CP may remain near 70; and for diffuse or bilateral damage vs. right damage decisions the % CP can hardly be expected to exceed 65" (Wheeler & Reitan, 1963, p. 699).

In the present study all four of the categories that Wheeler and Reitan used, controls, right, left and diffuse brain damage, were categorized in a single operation of keying. The results of this categorization operation are given in Table 11. Here 88.5% of the controls, 79.8% of right hemisphere cases, 80.8% of left hemisphere cases and 62.5% of diffuse cases were correctly predicted. These results were comparable to the results of the discriminant function cross validation study (Wheeler & Reitan, 1963). Also, since keying is a single operation a single measure of agreement can be obtained. Thus it can be concluded that a relatively simple process such as keying can obtain, in one operation, comparable results to the most sophisticated statistical method that must use many operations since it only handles binary groups of categories.

Evidently the reason for this advantage of the keying system as used here and by Meehl (1959) is that multiple decisions are utilized rather than a single one. No matter how complex the system of weighting when scores are combined, information is lost. Only a logical system, whether in the form of successive sieves (Wechsler, 1958), a hierarchically ordered sequential decision making model (Haynes & Sells, 1963), a set of rules (Meehl & Dahlstrom, 1960a), or a Key, can make decisions without combining scores and so losing information.

The Key, by cutting out the nonbrain damaged cases, initially eliminates them from the total pool thus preventing their scores from "washing out" other differences. These scores do not go into the pool to inflate the combined score. The information necessary to make the categorization is thus not "washed out."

Another way of stating this advantage of a Key is to describe the operation of indexes that do not combine the scores. Often in cases of brain damage not all of the tests administered are strongly influenced by the damage, so a combination of the scores will lose information. For instance, if the Key requires that only two scores need reach a severity scale score of 3 to indicate right hemisphere damage and the score results obtained are 0 1 3 2 4 1 1, the subject would be categorized as having right hemisphere damage. However, if these scores were averaged the combined criterion score is only 1.7. Of course, the cutting point might be lowered but this would increase the percentage of false inclusions.

Statistical procedures can and should eventually be combined with the logical keying method since obtaining every cutting point is essentially an actuarial procedure. It will be necessary to utilize statistics in many ways in constructing Keys, from investigating hypotheses that can later be added to a Key to determining cutting points.

In some cases the kind of statistics used will need to be different from those previously used by psychology; for instance, in the customary method of deriving cutting points, the point is set so as to reduce both false inclusions and false exclusions as much as possible. In a Key or any procedure that uses successive sieves the number of false inclusions initially is of no great importance since usually they will be eliminated by later sieves. The number of false exclusions, however, must be kept as low as possible since once a case is lost it cannot be regained.

Hathaway (1959) discusses this issue in a paper on increasing test efficiency. He points out that in most cases the percentage of false negatives is crucial, giving the example of a case in which a test indicator fails to identify a brain tumor. Even if the Key method did not tend to gradually eliminate false positives based on single indicators in predicting neurological diagnosis, the clinician may wish to stay on the safe side, even if this means generating a somewhat excessive number of false positives. Although this approach certainly should not be taken to extremes, it is still more desirable from the point of view of the patient's welfare to predict neurological disease when it is absent than not to predict it when it is present.

UTILITY OF KEYS

Keys have a considerable area of application. As used in psychology they consist of an objectification of inferential rules which neuropsychologists and clinicians have found helpful in diagnosing psychological entities. The sources for these rules can be either "soft" clinical ideas or "hard" verified hypotheses. As such it is an objective codification of the knowledge in an area of psychology. This characteristic gives the Key several kinds of practical application.

Practical Concerns

A major advantage of a Key is that it enables a clerk with little experience and training in a particular area to make accurate decisions in that area. In this study a rater with no formal knowledge of neuropsychology was able to categorize brain damaged patients essentially as accurately as an experienced neuropsychologist within the area of the Key's applicability. Since Keys can be improved through the use of statistical procedures and because they lack human variability and tendencies to forget, it is possible that eventually they will be more accurate than most psychologists dealing with their area of specialization. This appears to be true of the Meehl-Dahlstrom rules at present (Meehl, 1959).

It appears possible to program most Keys for a computer just as medical diagnosis can be programmed (Ledley & Lusted, 1959). Such programming, of course, adds accuracy and the ability to deal with large amounts of material. A computer program for the Keys used in the present study is presented in the appendix of this book. It might also often be convenient for a psychologist to have a book of Keys he can utilize to categorize some unfamiliar pattern of tests without the difficulty of sending single records to a computer center. Certainly, this way of using Keys has been the primary way that Keys have functioned for the biologist.

Education

Keys could serve several educational purposes. Since they contain the knowledge that previous experience and research have established, they constitute a teaching device. The Keys used in this study were designed with this function in mind.

Another educational advantage is that Keys will enable the inexperienced person who is establishing his own laboratory to attain an accuracy that would otherwise require much more experience. He would not have to build up an internal fund of knowledge, and mistakes, in order to make fairly accurate assessments within the area of the Key's capabilities.

Also, whenever any psychologist encounters a problem outside of his field of specialization he becomes an inexperienced person. A Key in that area would consequently improve his functioning. It would give him a greater range of effectiveness than he would have without the Key. In biology an expert may know all the species within a certain limited range but Keys are necessary for him to operate effectively outside that range.

Research

Keys can be helpful in research in several ways. First they can be used to integrate the results of research. In the Keys used in this study the results of a large number of research investigations were incorporated into an ordered form. Verified hypotheses may constitute the basis for a Key. In some cases a part of a Key that has not been thoroughly studied may prove to be an effective part. In this case the part can be used as the basis for a hypothesis. Thus Keys may be useful in forming hypotheses for further investigations. Kleinmuntz' (1963) method for collecting inferential rules, that is, by tape recording the vocalization of an expert while he was analyzing MMPI protocols, also constitutes fertile ground for growing research. In addition, extensive research, of course, is needed to determine the optimal cutting scores for each criteria.

Since the Key constitutes an objectification of the inferential process, it exteriorizes that process so that it can be studied, at least in its formal properties. This kind of research can be applied to the way psychologists think as diagnosticians, when they are thinking accurately, through placing their inferences into a Key format. Ledley and Lusted (1959) have demonstrated how the thinking used by physicians can be placed into a logical system. They did this by analyzing how physicians think while making a diagnosis. Consequently, studies can also be done on sources of the errors that clinicians make by comparing their thinking with Keys that give an accurate account of how thinking should proceed.

A General Psychological Method

Since valid Keys have been constructed for two areas of psychology, brain damage and MMPI profile analysis, it is evident that Keys could be produced in almost all areas of psychology in which reliable groups of tests are utilized or could be utilized. There is also the possibility that they could be applied to material which can either not be quantified or only crudely quantified. Clinical judgment might need to replace the objective scores in such Keys but the logic of the reasoning process could still be given in the form of a Key. In making Keys a tremendous amount of clinical experience, which might or might not be correct, could be placed in a testable form. Every Key statement can be viewed as a hypothesis to be evaluated in future research. Kleinmuntz' (1963) method of recording vocalized reasoning of expert clinicians and then transforming this reasoning into a set of rules placed in Key form would be particularly valuable in this regard. In conclusion it appears that the concept of a Key as an ordered set of rules for assessing and classifying psychological data could become a new method in psychology with a considerable area of application.

Bibliography

Andersen, A. L. The effect of laterality localization of brain damage on Wechsler-Bellevue indices of deterioration. *Journal of Clinical Psychology,* 1950, **6,** 191–194.

Armitage, S. G. An analysis of certain psychological tests used for the evaluation of brain injury. *Psychological Monographs,* 1946, **60** (1, Whole No. 277).

Bauer, R. W. & Wepman, J. M. Lateralization of cerebral functions. *Journal of Speech and Hearing Disorders,* 1955, **20,** 171–176.

Beckner, M. *The Biological Way of Thought.* New York: Columbia University Press, 1959.

Boring, E. G. *A History of Experimental Psychology.* New York: Appleton-Century-Crofts, 1950.

Bruell, J. H. & Albee, G. W. Higher intellectual functions in a patient with hemispherectomy for tumor. *Journal of Consulting Psychology,* 1962, **26,** 90–98.

Clements, F. E. & Clements, E. S. *Rocky Mountain Flowers.* New York: Wilson, 1945.

Cohen, J. The efficacy of diagnostic pattern analysis with the Wechsler-Bellevue. *Journal of Consulting Psychology,* 1955, **19,** 303–306.

Cohen, J. A coefficient of agreement for nominal scales. *Educational and Psychological Measurement,* 1960, **20,** 37–46.

Dahlstrom, W. G. & Welsh, G. S. *An MMPI Handbook.* Minneapolis: University of Minnesota Press, 1960.

Doehring, D. G., Reitan, R. M. & Kløve, H. Changes in patterns of intelligence test in brain-damaged patients with homonymous visual field defects. *AMA Archives of Neurology,* 1961, **5,** 294–299.

Doehring, D. G. & Reitan, R. M. Concept attainment of human adults with lateralized cerebral lesions. *Perceptual and Motor Skills,* 1962, **14,** 27–33.

Doehring, D. G., Reitan, R. M. & Kløve, H. Changes in patterns of intelligence test performance associated with homonymous visual field defects. *Journal of Nervous and Mental Diseases,* 1961, **123,** 227–233.

Elliott, H. C. *Textbook of Neuroanatomy.* Philadelphia: Lippincott, 1963.

Finney, J. C. Programmed interpretation of MMPI and CPI. *Archives of General Psychiatry,* 1966, **15,** 75–81.

Fitzhugh, K. B. & Fitzhugh, L. C. WAIS results for *S*s, with long standing chronic, lateralized and diffuse cerebral dysfunction. *Perceptual and Motor Skills,* 1964, **19,** 735–739. (a)

Fitzhugh, K. B., Fitzhugh, L. C. & Reitan, R. M. Psychological deficits in relation to acuteness of brain dysfunction. *Journal of Consulting Psychology,* 1961, **25,** 61–66.

Fitzhugh, K. B., Fitzhugh, L. C. & Reitan, R. M. Wechsler-Bellevue comparisons in groups with "chronic" and "current" lateralized and diffuse brain lesions. *Journal of Consulting Psychology,* 1962, **26,** 306–310. (a)

Fitzhugh, K. B., Fitzhugh, L. C. & Reitan, R. M. Relation of acuteness of organic brain dysfunction to trail-making test performances. *Perceptual and Motor Skills,* 1962, **15,** 399–403. (b)

Fitzhugh, L. C. & Fitzhugh, K. B. Relationships between Wechsler-Bellevue Form I and WAIS performances of subjects with long standing cerebral dysfunction. *Perceptual and Motor Skills,* 1964, **19,** 539–543. (b)

Gardner, W. J., Karnosh, L. J., McClure, C. C. & Gardner, A. K. Residual function following hemispherectomy for tumor and for infantile hemiplegia. *Brain,* 1955, **78,** 487–502.

Gazzaniga, M. S., Bogen, J. E. & Sperry, R. W. Observations on visual perception after disconnection of the cerebral hemispheres in man. *Brain,* 1965, **88,** 221–236.

Gazzaniga, M. S. & Sperry, R. W. Language after section of the cerebral commissures. *Brain,* 1967, **90,** 131–148.

Gilmore, J. S. L. Taxonomy and philosophy. In J. S. Huxley (Ed.), *The New Systematics*. Oxford: Clarendon Press, 1940, 461–474.

Gilmore, J. S. L. The development of taxonomic theory since 1851. *Nature,* 1951, **168,** 400–402.

Goldstein, K. *The Organism*. New York: American Book, 1939.

Goldstein, K. *Language and Language Disturbance*. New York: Grune & Stratton, 1948.

Goldstein, K. & Scheerer, M. Abstract and concrete behavior: An experimental study with special tests. *Psychological Monographs,* 1941, **53** (2, Whole No. 239).

Gough, H. C. Clinical versus statistical prediction in psychology. In L. Postman (Ed.), *Psychology in the Making*. New York: Knopf, 1962.

Graham, F. K. & Kendall, B. S. Memory-for-designs test: Revised general manual. *Perceptual and Motor Skills,* 1960, **11,** 147–188 (Monogr. Suppl. 2-VII).

Halstead, W. C. *Brain and Intelligence*. Chicago: University of Chicago Press, 1947.

Halstead, W. C. Biological intelligence. *Journal of Personality,* 1951, **20,** 118–130. (a)

Halstead, W. C. Brain and intelligence. In L. A. Jeffress (Ed.), *Cerebral Mechanisms in Behavior: The Hixon Symposium*. New York: Wiley, 1951, 244–272. (b)

Halstead, W. C. & Wepman, J. M. The Halstead-Wepman aphasia screening test. *Journal of Speech and Hearing Disorders,* 1949, **14,** 9–15.

Hathaway, S. R. A coding system for MMPI profiles. *Journal of Consulting Psychology,* 1947, **11,** 334–337.

Hathaway, S. R. Increasing clinical efficiency. In B. M. Bass & I. W. Berg (Eds.), *Objective Approaches to Personality Assessment*. New York: Van Nostrand, 1959.

Haynes, J. R. & Sells, S. B. Assessment of organic brain damage by psychological tests. *Psychological Bulletin,* 1963, **60,** 316–325.

Hebb, D. O. Intelligence in man after large removals of cerebral tissue: Defects following right temporal lobectomy. *Journal of General Psychology,* 1939, **21,** 437–446.

Hebb, D. O. *The Organization of Behavior*. New York: Wiley, 1949.

Heimburger, F. R. & Reitan, R. M. Easily administered written test for lateralizing brain lesions. *Journal of Neurosurgery,* 1961, **18,** 301–312.

Heinrichs, T. S. Objective configural rules for discriminating MMPI profiles in a psychiatric population. *Journal of Clinical Psychology,* 1964, **20,** 157–159.

Heinrichs, T. S. A note on the extension of MMPI configural rules. *Journal of Clinical Psychology,* 1966, **22,** 51–52.

Hewson, L. The Wechsler-Bellevue scale and substitution test as aids in neuropsychiatric diagnosis. *Journal of Nervous and Mental Diseases,* 1949, **109,** 158–266.

Holt, R. R. Clinical and statistical prediction: A reformulation and some new data. *Journal of Abnormal and Social Psychology,* 1958, **56,** 1–12.

Holt, R. R. & Luborsky, L. *Personality Patterns of Psychiatrists.* Vols. I & II. New York: Basic Books, 1958.

Kleinmuntz, B. Personality test interpretation by digital computer. *Science,* 1963, **139,** 416–418.

Kløve, H. The relationship of differential electroencephalographic patterns to distribution of Wechsler-Bellevue scores. *Neurology,* 1959, **9,** 871–876. (a)

Kløve, H. The relationship of sensory suppression to distribution of Wechsler-Bellevue scores. Paper presented at the meeting of the Midwestern Psychological Association, Chicago, May, 1959. (b)

Kløve, H. & Fitzhugh, K. B. The relationship of differential EEG patterns to the distribution of Wechsler-Bellevue scores in a chronic epileptic population. *Journal of Clinical Psychology,* 1962, **18,** 334–337.

Kløve, H. & Reitan, R. M. The effect of dysphasia and spatial distortion on Wechsler-Bellevue results. *AMA Archives of Neurology and Psychiatry,* 1958, **80,** 708–713.

Ladd, C. E. WAIS performance of brain damaged and neurotic patients. *Journal of Clinical Psychology,* 1964, **20,** 114–117.

Ledley, R. S. & Lusted, L. B. Reasoning foundation of medical diagnosis. *Science,* 1959, **130,** 9–21.

Lindzey, G. Seer versus sign. *Journal of Experimental Research in Personality,* 1965, **1,** 17–26.

Lykken, D. T. A method of actuarial pattern analysis. *Psychological Bulletin,* 1956, **53,** 102–107.

Marks, P. A. & Seeman, W. *The Actuarial Description of Abnormal Personality.* Baltimore: Williams & Wilkins, 1963.

Matthews, C. G., Guertin, W. H. & Reitan, R. M. Wechsler-Bellevue subtest mean rank orders in diverse diagnostic groups. *Psychological Reports,* 1962, **11,** 3–9.

Matthews, C. G. & Reitan, R. M. Correlations of Wechsler-Bellevue rank orders of subtest means in lateralized and non-lateralized brain damaged groups. *Perceptual and Motor Skills,* 1964, **19,** 391–394.

McDowell, F. & Wolff, H. G. *Handbook of Neurological Diagnostic Methods.* Baltimore: Williams & Wilkins, 1960.

Meehl, P. E. *Clinical versus Statistical Prediction.* Minneapolis: University of Minnesota Press, 1954.

Meehl, P. E. A comparison of clinicians with five statistical methods of identifying psychotic MMPI profiles. *Journal of Counseling Psychology,* 1959, **6,** 102–109.

Meehl, P. E. & Dahlstrom, W. G. Objective configural rules for discriminating psychotic from neurotic MMPI profiles. *Journal of Consulting Psychology,* 1960, **24,** 375–387. (a)

Meehl, P. E. & Dalstrom, W. G. Rules for profile discrimination, Appendix J. In W. C. Dalstrom & G. S. Welsh (Eds.) *An MMPI Handbook.* Minneapolis: University of Minnesota Press, 1960. (b)

Meehl, P. E. Seer over sign: the first good example. *Journal of Experimental Research in Personality,* 1965, **1,** 27–32.

Metcalf, Z. P. The construction of keys. *Systematic Zoology,* 1954, **3,** 38–45.

Mettler, F. A. (Ed.), *Selective Partial Ablation of the Frontal Cortex.* New York: Hoeber, 1949.

Mettler, F. A. (Ed.), *Psychosurgical Problems.* New York: Blaikeston, 1952.

Meyer, V. Psychological effects of brain damage. In H. J. Eysenck (Ed.), *Handbook of Abnormal Psychology.* New York: Basic Books, 1961, 529–565.

Milner, B. Psychological defects produced by temporal lobe excision. In H. C. Soloman, S. Cobb & W. Penfield (Eds.), *The Brain and Human Behavior.* Baltimore: Williams & Wilkins, 1956, 244–257.

Milner, B. Laterality effects in audition. In V. B. Mountcastle (Ed.), *Interhemispheric Relations and Cerebral Dominance.* Baltimore: Johns Hopkins University Press, 1962, 177–195.

Penfield, W. Speech, perception and the cortex. In J. C. Eccles (Ed.), *Brain and Conscious Experience.* New York: Springer-Verlag, 1966, 217–237.

Penfield, W. & Roberts, L. *Speech and Brain Mechanisms.* Princeton, New York: Princeton University Press, 1959.

Piercy, M. The effects of cerebral lesions on intellectual function: A review of current research trends. *British Journal of Psychiatry,* 1964, **110,** 310–352.

Piotrowski, Z. A. Digital-computer interpretation of inkblot test data. *Psychiatric Quarterly,* 1964, **38**(1), 1–26.

Pribram, K. H. Interrelations of psychology and the neurological disciplines. In S. Koch, *Psychology: A Study of a Science,* Vol. 4. New York: McGraw-Hill, 1962, 119–157.

Reed, H. B. C. & Reitan, R. M. Intelligence test performances of brain-damaged subjects with lateralized motor deficits. *Journal of Consulting Psychology,* 1963, **27,** 102–106.

Reitan, R. M. Certain differential effects of left and right cerebral lesions in human adults. *Journal of Comparative* and *Physiologicol and Psychology,* 1955, **48,** 474–477. (a)

Reitan, R. M. Investigation of the validity of Halstead's measures of biological intelligence. *Archives of Neurology and Psychiatry,* 1955, **48,** 474–477. (b)

Reitan, R. M. The relation of the Trail Making Test to organic brain damage. *Journal of Consulting Psychology,* 1955, **19,** 393–394. (c)

Reitan, R. M. Investigation of relationships between "psychometric" and "biological" intelligence. *Journal of Nervous and Mental Diseases,* 1956, **123,** 536–541.

Reitan, R. M. The comparative significance of qualitative and quantitative psychological changes with brain damage. *Proceedings of Fifteenth International Congress of Psychology,* 1957, 214–215.

Reitan, R. M. Qualitative versus quantitative mental changes following brain damage. *Journal of Psychology,* 1958, **46,** 339–346. (a)

Reitan, R. M. Symposium: Contributions of physiological psychology to clinical inferences. Paper presented at the meeting of the Midwestern Psychological Association, Detroit, May, 1958. (b)

Reitan, R. M. The validity of the Trail Making Test as an indicator of organic brain damage. *Perceptual and Motor Skills,* 1958, **8,** 271–276. (c)

Reitan, R. M. The comparative effects of brain damage on the Halstead Impairment Index and the Wechsler-Bellevue scale. *Journal of Clinical Psychology,* 1959, **15,** 281–285. (a)

Reitan, R. M. The effects of brain damage on a psychomotor problem-solving task. *Perceptual and Motor Skills,* 1959, **9,** 211–215. (b)

Reitan, R. M. The effects of brain lesions on adaptive abilities in human beings. Unpublished Monograph, 1959. (c)

Reitan, R. M. Impairment of abstraction ability in brain damage: Qualitative versus quantitative changes. *Journal of Psychology,* 1959, **48,** 97–102. (d)

Reitan, R. M. The significance of dysphasia for intelligence and adaptive abilities. *Journal of Psychology,* 1960, **50,** 355–376.

Reitan, R. M. Psychological deficit. *Annual Review of Psychology,* 1962, **13,** 415–444.

Reitan, R. M. Psychological deficits resulting from cerebral lesions in man. In J. M. Warren & K. Akert (Eds.), *The Frontal Granular Cortex and Behavior.* New York: McGraw-Hill, 1964, 295–312. (a)

Reitan, R. M. Relationships between neurological and psychological variables and their implications for reading instruction. In H. A. Robinson (Ed.), *Meeting Individual Differences in Reading.* Chicago: University of Chicago Press, 1964, 100–110. (b)

Reitan, R. M. A research program on the psychological effects of brain lesions in human beings. In N. R. Ellis (Ed.), *International Review of Research in Mental Retardation,* Vol. I. New York: Academic Press, 1966, pp. 153–218.

Semmes, J. Weinstein, S., Ghent, L. & Teuber, H. L. Correlates of impaired orientation in personal and extra-personal space. *Brain,* 1963, **86,** 747–772.

Shaw, D. J. The reliability and validity of the Halstead Category test. *Journal of Clinical Psychology,* 1966, **22,** 176–179.

Shure, G. H. & Halstead, W. C. Cerebral localization of intellectual processes. *Psychological Monographs,* 1958, **72** (Whole No. 465).

Siegel, S. *Nonparametric Statistics for the Behavioral Sciences.* New York: McGraw-Hill, 1956.

Smith, A. Ambiguities in concepts and studies of "brain damage" and "organicity." *Journal of Nervous and Mental Diseases,* 1962, **135,** 311–326. (a)

Smith, A. Psychodiagnosis of patients with brain tumors: The validity of Hewson's ratios in neurology and mental hospital populations. *Journal of Nervous and Mental Diseases,* 1962, **135,** 513–533. (b)

Smith, A. & Burklund, C. W. Dominant hemispherectomy: Preliminary report on neuropsychological sequelae. *Science,* 1966, **153,** 1280–1282.

Sneath, P. H. A. The construction of taxonomic groups. In G. C. Ainsworth & P. H. A. Sneath (Eds.), *Microbial Classification,* 12th Symposium of the Society for General Microbiology, Cambridge: Cambridge University Press, 1962, 289–332.

Sokal, R. R. & Sneath, P. H. *Principles of Numerical Taxonomy.* San Francisco: Freeman, 1963.

Sperry, R. W. Cerebral organization and behavior. *Science,* 1961, **133,** 1749–1757.

Sullivan, P. L. & Welsh, G. S. A technique for objective configural analysis of MMPI profiles. *Journal of Consulting Psychology,* 1952, **16,** 383–388.

Talland, G. A. Psychology's concern with brain damage. *Journal of Nervous and Mental Diseases,* 1963, **136,** 344–351.

Taulbee, E. C. & Sissons, B. D. Configural analysis of MMPI profiles of psychiatric groups. *Journal of Consulting Psychology,* 1957, **21,** 413–417.

Teuber, H. L. Effects of brain wounds implicating right or left hemisphere in man: Hemisphere differences and hemisphere interaction in vision, audition and somesthesis. In E. B. Mountcastle (Ed.), *Interhemispheric Relations and Cerebral Dominance.* Baltimore: Johns Hopkins University Press, 1962, 131–157.

Teuber, H. L. Alterations of perception after brain injury. In J. C. Eccles (Ed.), *Brain and Conscious Experience,* New York: Springer-Verlag, 1966, 182–216.

van Wagener, W. P. & Harren, R. Y. Surgical divisions of commissural pathways in the corpus collosum. *Archives of Neurology and Psychiatry,* 1940, **44,** 740–759.

Voss, E. G. The history of keys and phylogenetic trees in systematic biology. *Journal of the Scientific Laboratory of Denison University,* 1952, **43,** 1–25.

Warrington, E. K. & James, M. Disorders of visual perception in patients with localized cerebral lesions. *Neuropsychologia,* 1967, **5,** 253–266.

Wechsler, D. *The Measurement of Adult Intelligence,* 3rd Edition. Baltimore: Williams & Wilkins, 1944.

Wechsler, D. *The Measurement and Appraisal of Adult Intelligence,* 4th Edition. Baltimore: Williams & Wilkins, 1958.

Weinstein, S. & Teuber, H. L. Effects of penetrating brain injury on intelligence test scores. *Science,* 1957, **125,** 1036–1037.

Wheeler, L. Predictions of brain damage from an aphasia screening test; An application of discriminant functions and a comparison with a non-linear method of analysis. *Perceptual and Motor Skills,* 1963, **17,** 63–80.

Wheeler, L., Burke, C. J. & Reitan, R. M. An application of discriminant functions to the problem of predicting brain damage using behavioral variables. *Perceptual and Motor Skills,* 1963, **16,** 417–440 (Monogr. Suppl. 3-V16).

Wheeler, L. & Reitan, R. M. The presence and laterality of brain damage predicted from responses to a short aphasia screening test. *Perceptual and Motor Skills,* 1962, **15,** 783–799.

Wheeler, L. & Reitan, R. M. Discriminant functions applied to the problems of predicting cerebral damage from behavioral tests; a cross validation study. *Perceptual and Motor Skills,* 1963, **16,** 681–701.

Williamson, E. B. Keys in systematic work. *Science,* 1922, **55,** 703–713.

Wolff, B. B. The application of Hewson ratios as an aid in differential diagnosis of cerebral pathology. *Journal of Nervous and Mental Diseases,* 1960, **130,** 98–109.

APPENDIX A

Revised Norms for Rating Equivalents of Raw Scores

Revised Norms for Rating Equivalents of Raw Scores

Test	Rating Equivalents of Raw Scores					
	0	1	2	3	4	5
Average Impairment Rating	0.00–1.00	1.01–1.35	1.36–2.00	2.01–2.85	2.86–3.50	3.51–5.00
Category errors	≤25	26–52	53–75	76–105	106–131	132+
(TPT) Time						
Dominant hand	≤4.7	4.8–8.2	8.3–10	10 min. and 9–5 blocks	10 min. and 4–2 blocks	10 min. and 1–0 blocks
Nondominant hand	≤2.6	2.7–4.5	4.6–6.1	6.2–8.8	8.9–10 and 10–6 blocks	10 min. and 5–0 blocks
Both hands	≤1.5	1.6–2.7	2.8–3.7	3.8–5.2	5.3–10	10 min. and 9–0 blocks
Total	≤9.0	9.1–15.6	15.7–21	21.1–29.9	30 min. and 14–30 blocks	30 min. and 13–0 blocks
(TPT) Memory (No. correct)	10–9	8–6	5–4	3–2	1	0
(TPT) Location (No. correct)	10–7	6–5	4–3	2–1	0 and TPT Memory > 0	0 and TPT Memory = 0

Rhythm errors	0–2	3–5	6–9	10–13	14–18	19+
Speech errors	0–3	4–7	8–14	15–25	26–30	31+
Tapping (No.)						
Dom M	⩾55	54–50	49–43	42–32	31–20	19–0
F	⩾51	50–46	45–39	38–28	27–16	15–0
Nondom M	⩾49	48–44	43–37	36–26	25–14	13–0
F	⩾45	44–40	39–33	32–22	21–10	9–0
Trails A (time)	⩽19	20–33	34–48	49–62	63–86	87+
Trails B (time)	⩽57	58–87	88–123	124–186	187–275	276+
Aphasia (errors)	0	1–6	7–15	16–25	26–40	41+
Spatial Relations (errors)	1	2–3	4–5	6–7	8–9	10–12
Perceptual (errors)	0–4	5–12	13–30	31–50	51–80	81+
Visual suppression						
One eye	0	1	2	3	4	5
Two eyes	0	1–2	3–4	5–6	7–8	9–10
Heminaopia (count fields not eyes)	⩾191	190–121	120–97	96–73	72–47	48–0
		(invalid if total number of functioning squares in both eyes is ⩽96).				
Digit symbol $(Av - 1) = \frac{PA + PC + BD}{3} - 1$	DS⩾12 and ⩾(Av−1)	DS⩾12 and <(Av−1) or DS=9–11 DS=7–8 and ⩾(Av−1)	DS=7–8 and <(Av−1) or DS=5–6 and ⩾(Av−1)	DS=5–6 and <(Av−1) or DS=3–4 and ⩾(Av−1)	DS=3–4 and <(Av−1) or DS=2–1 and ⩾(Av−1)	DS=2–0 and <(Av−1)

APPENDIX B

Scoring for Aphasia

SCORING RULES FOR VERBAL SECTION

A. Count correct

1. An immediate recovery; for example, "I don't know, a cross I reckon."
2. If part of a word is given but corrected; for example, "Dia—triangle."
3. A simple confusion of instructions with correction, saying a response instead of writing, then writing it correctly.
4. Regardless of mispronunciation (except items 18, 19, 20 of the Aphasia Screening Test).
5. Lack of capitalization.
6. If the error is evidently due to misunderstanding of instructions.

B. Count incorrect

1. Any wrong word even with recovery.
2. Any extended hesitation.
3. Any circumlocution; for example, "It has corners—guess you could call it a square."
4. Any substitution of words in written or repeated sentences no matter how trivial; for example, substituting "a" for "the."
5. Mispronunciation in 18, 19, 20.

Rating Equivalents

Scores,	0	1–6	7–15	16–25	26–40	41+
Ratings,	0	1	2	3	4	5

APHASIA SCREENING-TEST

NAME ________________ DATE ____________ EXAMINER ____________

C&T = Comments, techniques, etc.

Copy SQUARE (C&T)

Name SQUARE

4

Spell SQUARE

1

Copy CROSS (C&T)

Name CROSS

4

Spell CROSS

1

Copy TRIANGLE (C&T)

Name TRIANGLE

2

Spell TRIANGLE

1

Name BABY

Write CLOCK (C&T)

3

Name FORK

4

Read 7 SIX 2

3

Read M G W

3

Read SEE THE BLACK DOG

2

Read HE IS A FRIENDLY ANIMAL A FAMOUS WINNER OF DOG SHOWS

1

Repeat TRIANGLE

1

Repeat MASSACHUSETTS

1

Repeat METHODIST EPISCOPAL

Item	Score	Item	Score
Write SQUARE	4	Compute 17 x 3 =	1
Read SEVEN	3	8 x 6 =	2
Repeat SEVEN	3	3 x 4 =	
Repeat HE SHOUTED THE WARNING	4	Name KEY	
Expalin HE SHOUTED THE WARNING	4	Demonstrate the use of KEY	4
Write HE SHOUTED THE WARNING	2 or 4	Draw KEY (C&T)	4
Compute 85 − 27 =	2	Read PLACE LEFT HAND TO RIGHT EAR	
48 − 25 =	2	Place LEFT HAND TO RIGHT EAR	2
9 − 6 =		Place LEFT HAND TO LEFT ELBOW	2
			3

Total Error Score____________

Score for Best Cross____________

Score for Worst Cross____________

APPENDIX C

Scoring for Spatial Relations

On the Aphasia Examination the subject is asked to draw at least two Greek crosses. These drawings are to be compared with the examples on the following pages. Each cross is given a score of 1 to 5, depending upon which of the examples it most resembles. If more than two crosses were drawn, count the best one and the worst one.

If WAIS Block Design is the lowest (not equal) scale score except for Digit Symbol and Object Assembly, add two points to the total score for the two crosses; this is the total Spatial Relations Score. If Block Design is not the lowest scale score except for Digit Symbol and Object Assembly, the total Spatial Relations Score is the sum of the two cross scores.

Rating Equivalents

Scores,	1	2–3	4–5	6–7	8–9	10–12
Ratings,	0	1	2	3	4	5

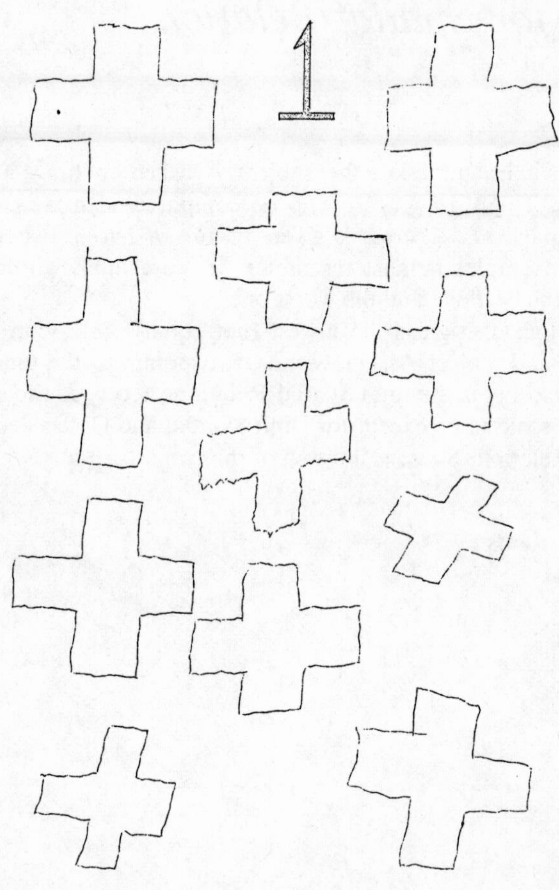

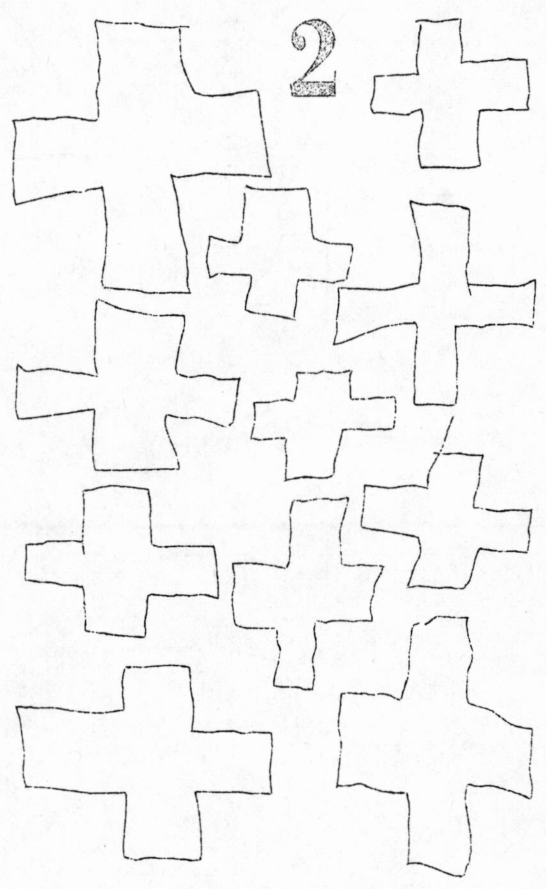
2

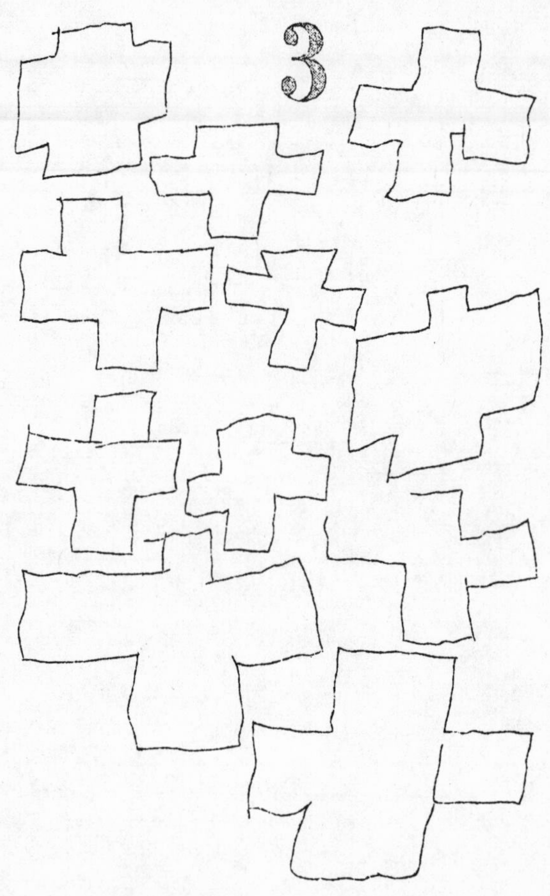
3

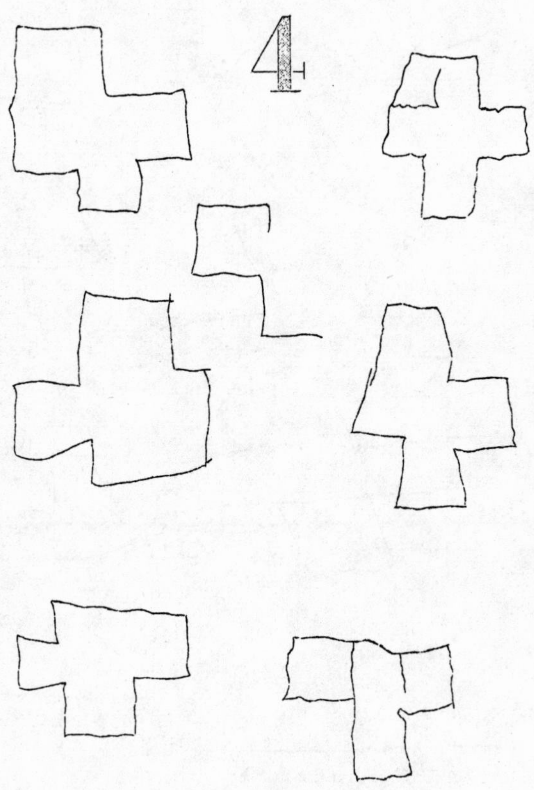

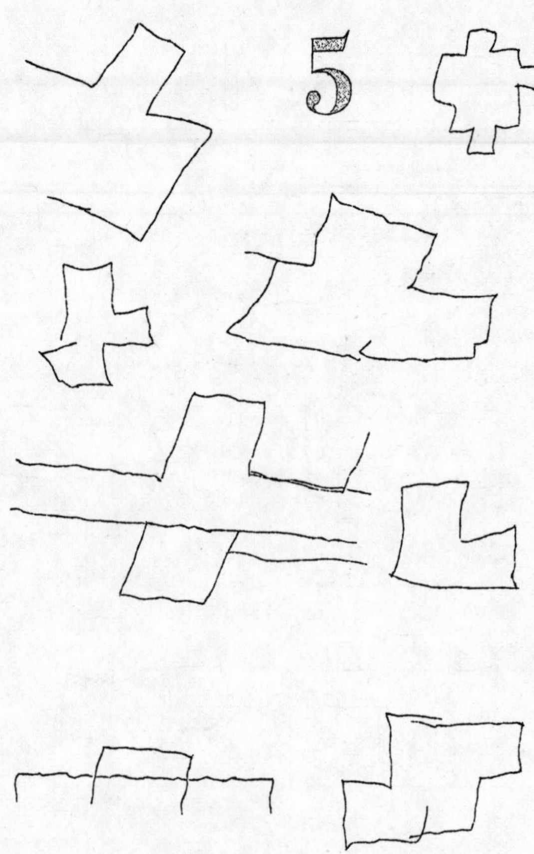
5

APPENDIX D

Scoring for Perceptual Disorders

SCORE ONLY

Suppressions, Finger Agnosia errors and Fingertip Writing errors.

SUPPRESSION (Double simultaneous stimulation: Tactile, Auditory, and Visual)

To score this count all errors in all modalities and then add half of that number (round up). If single stimulation shows a loss of 3 or 4 in any part of a modality such as RH or RUV do not count suppression in that part of the modality (or if threshold on Von Frey hair is number ≥ 7); for example, subject 152 has no vision in his left eye so do not score the whole visual area. His score for suppression should be $6 + 3 = 9$. His total score is 27.

FINGER AGNOSIA AND FINGERTIP WRITING

Always count errors made with both hands unless *S* has only one hand.

Rating Equivalents

Scores,	0–4	5–12	13–30	31–50	51–	81+
Ratings,	0	1	2	3	4	5

PERCEPTUAL DISORDERS

PERCEPTUAL DISORDERS

NAME________________ DATE__________ EXAMINER__________

KEY: X = not tested; dash = normal; # = number of errors. For Tests II through V, ratings are entered on asterisked (*) lines.
RATING SYSTEM: dash = normal; 1 = questionable; 2 = mild dysfunction; 3 = moderate dysfunction; 4 = severe dysfunction.

Single Stimulation | **Double Stimulation**

I. TACTILE

Threshold	R-L Errors	Both	Threshold	L-R Errors	Both
RH Hair No___	RH___#	RH___#	LH Hair No___	LH___#	LH___#
RF Hair No___	RF___#	RF___#	LF Hair No___	LF___#	LF___#

Circle Suppressed Side

	Trials 1	2	3	4	Both
RH-LH	R-L	R-L	R-L	R-L	
RH-LF	R-L	R-L	R-L	R-L	
RF-LH	R-L	R-L	R-L	R-L	

II. AUDITORY
Audiometry (if available): RE___% LE___% Combined___%

Loss	R-L Confusion	Both	Loss	L-R Confusion	Both
RE___*	RE___#	RE___#	LE___*	LE___#	LE___#

Circle Suppressed Side

	Trials 1	2	3	4	Both
RE-LE	R-L	R-L	R-L	R-L	

III. VISUAL (Fields: 1. Normal: ____
2. Abnormal: ________)

Miss	Confusion	Both	Miss	Confusion	Both
RUV___*	RUV___#	RUV___#	LUV___*	LUV___#	LUV___#
RMV___*	RMV___#	RMV___#	LMV___*	LMV___#	LMV___#
RLV___*	RLV___#	RLV___#	LLV___*	LLV___#	LLV___#

Circle Suppressed Side

	Trials 1	2	3	4	Both
RUV-LUV	R-L	R-L	R-L	R-L	
RMV-LMV	R-L	R-L	R-L	R-L	
RLV-LLV	R-L	R-L	R-L	R-L	

IV. FINGER AGNOSIA

	1	2	3	4	5	Error
Right:	1	2	3	4	5	/
Left:	1	2	3	4	5	/

V. FINGER-TIP NUMBER WRITING:

	4 6 3 5	3 5 4 6	6 5 4 3	5 4 6 3	6 3 5 4	Error
Right:	1	2	3	4	5	/
Left:	1	2	3	4	5	/

APPENDIX E

Scoring for Lateral Dominance Scale

To be applied to the Lateral Dominance Examination used in Reitan's Neuropsychological Laboratory (see next page).

For the hand dominance measure use part No. 2; first seven items. Count each item as 1 except for "write your name" which is scored as 3. If "both" is scored, give .5 to each hand. For the eye dominance measure use the Miles ABC, all 10 picture cards.

Mixed Dominance measure (right versus left hand) score as mixed if any of these ratios occur: 6:3, 5:4, 4:5, 3:6; for example, if right hand is 3 and left is 6, score as mixed.

Crossed Dominance measure (dominant hand to opposite eye) score as crossed if dominant hand is 9, 8 or 7 and the opposite eye is 10, 9, 8 or 7; for example, if right hand is 9 and left eye is 8, score as crossed dominance.

LATERAL DOMINANCE EXAMINATION

Project #360
Neuropsychology

______

LATERAL DOMINANCE EXAMINATION

NAME______________________________ DATE_______________ EXAMINER________________

1. Show me your: right hand_____ left ear_____ right eye_____

2. Show me how you:

	B	R	L
throw a ball			
hammer a nail			
cut with a knife			
turn a door knob			
use scissors			
use an eraser			
write your name			
TOTAL			

fold your hands_______ top thumb
fold your arms _______ tucked arm

3. Write full name: DH ( )_______ secs. NDH ( )_______ secs.

Write TELEVISION: DH _______ secs. NDH _______ secs.

4. Strength of grip: (hold dynamometer at arm's length, point to floor, and squeeze as hard as you can)

(1) DH ( )_______kg. (2) NDH ( )_______kg.

(3) DH ( )_______kg. (4) NDH ( )_______kg.

TOTAL_______kg. TOTAL_______kg.

____HAND MEAN_______kg. ____HAND MEAN_______kg.

5. Show me how you:

kick a football_______foot B_______
step on a bug_______foot R_______
cross your legs_______top leg L_______

6. ABC

(1)_____ (2)_____ (3)_____ (4)_____ (5)_____

(6)_____ (7)_____ (8)_____ (9)_____ (10)_____

7. Conclusions:

	Strongly L	Mainly L	Mixed	Mainly R	Strongly R
Hand					
Foot					
Eye					

APPENDIX F

Interim Summary[1]

10/11/65

I. ADMINISTRATIVE DATA

The patient is a 56-year-old male and former accountant who was admitted to this hospital for the first time on 8/16/65 as a transfer from VAH . . .

II. PROGRESS AND TREATMENT

The patient's difficulties first began in December of 1964 when he began to experience some impairment in the functioning of his legs. He was hospitalized at . . . for one week in March of 1965. The diagnosis at that time was amyotrophic lateral sclerosis. He was again hospitalized from May 19, 1965, to June 8, 1965, at . . . Pneumoencephalogram at that time demonstrated findings of cerebral and cerebellar atrophy. Following that hospitalization there was a gradual but noticeable progression in his neurological difficulties. On June 8, 1965, he was admitted to VA Hospital, . . . and then transferred to this hospital on 8/15/65.

On 9/8/65 the patient was examined by the neurological consultant, Dr. Foster, at which time he felt that the patient might well have a brain tumor and suggested the possibility of it being an acoustic neuroma. He advised that further diagnostic studies were indicated and the patient was forthwith transferred to VAH, ... At the time of his admission to that facility he had bilateral papilledema. The patient was seen to be alert, cooperative, but slightly confused and disoriented. He was unable to stand without assistance. With assistance the stance was wide-based and with marked instability. His cranial nerves were grossly intact. The patient did have a

[1]This neurological report has been abbreviated so as to retain only the information used to determine the location and process stage of the cerebral damage. Identifying information has also been removed.

slight left hemiparesis most marked in the arm. A slight hyperreflexia on the left was present with a positive left Babinski sign and a left ankle clonus. Following his admission a brain scan was done and a positive focus in the right cerebellar pontine angle was demonstrated. Consultation with an otolaryngologist provided further confirmation of the diagnosis of an acoustic neuroma on the right side. On 9/14/65 a right sub-occipital craniotomy was done with total removal of the acoustic neuroma. Post operatively the patient initially did well but then had a left-sided focal seizure beginning in the left hand. . . .

III. CONCLUSIONS

A. Diagnoses

1. Acoustic neuroma, right, post operative, improved. 2. VII, VIII, IX, and X cranial nerve damage on the right. 3. Right sub-occipital craniotomy defect. 4. Chronic brain syndrome associated with intracranial tumor, acoustic neuroma. 5. Diabetes mellitus, mild, treated, improved. 6. Pulmonary emphysema. 7. Bilateral pes planus.

Present Status of SCD: See Dg. 7.

B. Prognosis

A return in function of the injured cranial nerves may or may not occur; some return in function can be hoped for by the use of physical therapy and speech therapy. The therapeutic problems of greatest concern at this point, however, are with the treatment of the patient's tendency toward respiratory acidosis and to guard against infection—via the craniotomy site.

C. Competency

The patient is incompetent to handle VA funds.

No. 180 Neurological Service
VAH, Topeka, Kansas

NEUROLOGICAL AND NEUROPSYCHOLOGICAL EXAMINATION CHECK SHEET

Brain Damage: Localization

Neurological (X) Date: 8/17/87

Neuropsychological ( ) Scorer: ER

Case Name: —— Case No.: 140

No Brain Damage ( )

Possible Brain Damage ( )

Brain Damaged (X)

Lateralized Right (X)

R. Frontal ( )

R. Central ( )

R. Posterior (X) if any cortical damage is present

R. Undetermined ( )

Lateralized Left ( )

L. Frontal ( )

L. Central ( )

L. Posterior ( )

L. Undetermined ( )

Prefrontal ( )

Diffuse ( )

Undetermined Laterality ( )

Comments:

Tumor brain scan R cerebellar pontine angle — possibly peripheral nerve damage tested preoperatively

NEUROLOGICAL AND NEUROPSYCHOLOGICAL EXAMINATION CHECK SHEET

Brain Damage: Process

Neurological (X) Date: 9/17/67

Neuropsychological ( ) Scorer: Ek

Case Name: ______ Case No.: 140

No Brain Damage ( )

Possible Brain Damage ( )

Brain Damaged (X)

- Acute b.d. (under 3 months) (X)
- Static b.d. (over 1 year) ( )
- Congenital b.d. ( )
- Intermediate b.d. ( )
- Undetermined other ( )

Comments:

active tumor (acoustic neuroma)
at time of testing

Neuropsychology Data

September 8, 1965

This patient is severely impaired in almost all abilities tested, and appears to be suffering from an active, serious, diffuse neurological disease. While bilateral involvement is clearly indicated, there is some evidence that the right cerebral hemisphere is functioning less well than the left. In addition to his intellectual impairment, there is severe sensory, perceptual, and motor defect. His visual fields are somewhat constricted, showing some suggestion of tunnel vision.

The severe impairment demonstrated by this patient suggests the presence of a relatively recently acquired disease, probably neoplastic in nature. While severe MS can give a similar picture, the extensiveness of the deficit makes a tumor more likely. It would probably be of the infiltrating type, possibly a glioma.

GERALD GOLDSTEIN, Ph.D.
Staff Psychologist

No. 180
VA Hospital
Topeka, Kansas

NEUROLOGICAL AND NEUROPSYCHOLOGICAL EXAMINATION CHECK SHEET

Brain Damage: Localization

Neurological ( ) Date: 10/11/67

Neuropsychological (X) Scorer: CM

Case Name: ________ Case No.: 140

No Brain Damage ( )

Possible Brain Damage ( )

Brain Damaged (X)

- Lateralized Right ( )
  - R. Frontal ( )
  - R. Central ( )
  - R. Posterior ( )
  - R. Undetermined (X)
- Lateralized Left ( )
  - L. Frontal ( )
  - L. Central ( )
  - L. Posterior ( )
  - L. Undetermined ( )
- Prefrontal ( )
- Diffuse ( )
- Undetermined Laterality ( )

Comments:

NEUROLOGICAL AND NEUROPSYCHOLOGICAL EXAMINATION CHECK SHEET

Brain Damage: Process

Neurological ( ) Date: 10/11/67

Neuropsychological (X) Scorer: ER

Case Name: ______________ Case No.: 180

No Brain Damage ( )

Possible Brain. Damage ( )

Brain Damage (X)

- Acute b.d. (under 3 months) (X)
- Static b.d. (over 1 year) ( )
- Congenital b.d. ( )
- Intermediate b.d. ( )
- Undetermined other ( )

Comments:

Example 1

NEUROPSYCHOLOGICAL KEY

Summary Sheet

Case Name: — Case No. 180

Scorer: Jm Date: 3/11/67

TEST	SCORE	
Average Impairment Rating	4.17	0 1 2 3 4 (5) X
Basic Ratings		
Halstead Categories (total errors)	136	0 1 2 3 4 (5) X
TPT Time (total) T: 30.0 Bl: 0	—	0 1 2 3 4 (5) X
TPT Memory	1	0 1 2 3 (4) 5 X
TPT Location	0	0 1 2 3 (4) 5 X
Rhythm	16	0 1 2 3 (4) 5 X
Speech	21	0 1 2 (3) 4 5 X
Tapping (worst hand) L. (R.)	25	0 1 2 3 (4) 5 X
Trails B	300	0 1 2 3 4 (5) X
Digit Symbol	0	0 1 2 3 4 (5) X
Aphasia	4	0 (1) 2 3 4 5 X
Spatial Relations 10 + BD 2	12	0 1 2 3 4 (5) X
Perceptual Disorders (total)	97	0 1 2 3 4 (5) X
Additional Ratings		
Trails A	172	0 1 2 3 4 (5) X
TPT Time R T: 10.0 Bl: 0	—	0 1 2 3 4 (5) X
TPT Time L T: 10.0 Bl: 0	—	0 1 2 3 4 (5) X
Tapping R ((Dom.) Non-Dom.)	25	0 1 2 3 (4) 5 X
Tapping L (Dom. (Non-Dom.))	25	0 1 2 3 (4) 5 X
Finger Agnosia R	17	0 1 2 3 4 5 X
Finger Agnosia L	14	0 1 2 3 4 5 X
Finger Tip Writing R	15	0 1 2 3 4 5 X
Finger Tip Writing L	15	0 1 2 3 4 5 X
Tactile Hypesthesia R H (worst): — F: —	—	0 1 2 3 4 5 X
Tactile Hypesthesia L H (worst): — F: —	—	0 1 2 3 4 5 X
Suppression Tactile (total) R	6	0 1 2 3 4 5 X
Suppression Tactile (total) L	6	0 1 2 3 4 5 X
Suppression auditory R	0	0 1 2 3 4 5 X
Suppression auditory L	0	0 1 2 3 4 5 X
Suppression visual (total) R	2	0 1 2 3 4 5 X
Suppression visual (total) L	6	0 1 2 3 4 5 X
Homonymous Hemianopia R	137	0 1 2 3 4 5 X
Homonymous Hemianopia L	152	0 1 2 3 4 5 X

Date 3/11/67 Case No. 180

WAIS Age: 56 — IQ Equivalent

	IQ Equivalent	
$\frac{V + D + S}{3}$ (11, 10, 5) = 26⅔ X 6 = 52	96	
		Difference 31
$\frac{BD + OA}{2}$ (2, 2) = 2 X 5 = 10	65	
WAIS Verbal IQ	100	
WAIS Performance IQ	68	
Difference	32	
WAIS Full Scale IQ	86	

Dominance, Hand R 9 L 0 Mixed Dom. ___

Dominance, Eye R 9 L 1 Crossed Dom.___

NEUROPSYCHOLOGICAL KEY CHECK SHEET

Brain Damage: Localization (A)

Case Name: ____________________ Date: 11/3/67

Case No: 180

Scorer: Jm

No Brain Damage ( )

Possible Brain Damage ( )

Brain Damage (✓)

Lateralized Right (✓)

Lateralized Left ( )

Prefrontal ( )

Diffuse ( )

Comments:

NEUROPSYCHOLOGICAL KEY CHECK SHEET

Brain Damage: Process (C)

Date: 11/3/67

Case Name: ______________ Case No: 180

Scorer: jm

No Brain Damage ( )

Possible Brain Damage ( )

Brain Damaged (✓)

Acute Brain Damage (✓)

Type Unknown (1) ( )

Static Brain Damage (1) ( )

Type Unknown (2) ( )

Static Brain Damage (2) ( )

Type Unknown (3) ( )

Static Brain Damage (3) ( )

Congenital Brain Damage ( )

Comments:

Appendix G NEUROPSYCHOLOGICAL KEY
Example 2

Summary Sheet

Case Name: ——— Case No. 154

Scorer: JM Date: 1/11/67

TEST	SCORE	
Average Impairment Rating	1.25	0 (1) 2 3 4 5 X
Basic Ratings		
Halstead Categories (total errors)	19	(0) 1 2 3 4 5 X
TPT Time (total) T: 13.7 Bl: 30	—	0 (1) 2 3 4 5 X
TPT Memory	7	0 (1) 2 3 4 5 X
TPT Location	3	0 1 (2) 3 4 5 X
Rhythm	3	0 (1) 2 3 4 5 X
Speech	1	0 (1) 2 3 4 5 X
Tapping (worst hand) L. (R.)	46	0 1 (2) 3 4 5 X
Trails B	83	0 (1) 2 3 4 5 X
Digit Symbol	7	0 1 (2) 3 4 5 X
Aphasia	1	0 (1) 2 3 4 5 X
Spatial Relations 2 + BD 0	2	0 (1) 2 3 4 5 X
Perceptual Disorders (total)	16	0 1 (2) 3 4 5 X
Additional Ratings		
Trails A	47	0 1 (2) 3 4 5 X
TPT Time R T: 6.4 Bl: 10	—	0 (1) 2 3 4 5 X
TPT Time L T: 4.3 Bl: 10	—	0 (1) 2 3 4 5 X
Tapping R ((Dom.) Non-Dom.)	46	0 1 (2) 3 4 5 X
Tapping L (Dom. (Non-Dom.))	45	0 (1) 2 3 4 5 X
Finger Agnosia R	0	0 1 2 3 4 5 X
Finger Agnosia L	0	0 1 2 3 4 5 X
Finger Tip Writing R	1	0 1 2 3 4 5 X
Finger Tip Writing L	2	0 1 2 3 4 5 X
Tactile Hypesthesia R H (worst): — F: —	0	0 1 2 3 4 5 X
Tactile Hypesthesia L H (worst): — F: —	0	0 1 2 3 4 5 X
Suppression Tactile (total) R	1	0 1 2 3 4 5 X
Suppression Tactile (total) L	1	0 1 2 3 4 5 X
Suppression auditory R	0	0 1 2 3 4 5 X
Suppression auditory L	2	0 1 2 3 4 5 X
Suppression visual (total) R	0	0 1 2 3 4 5 X
Suppression visual (total) L	5	0 1 2 3 4 5 X
Homonymous Hemianopia R	165	0 1 2 3 4 5 X
Homonymous Hemianopia L	169	0 1 2 3 4 5 X

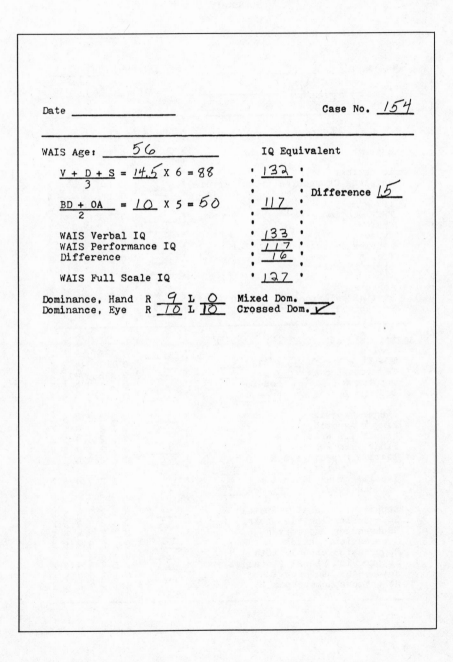

Date ______________ Case No. 154

WAIS Age: 56 IQ Equivalent

$\frac{V + D + S}{3}$ = 14.5 X 6 = 88 : 132 :

Difference 15

$\frac{BD + OA}{2}$ = 10 X 5 = 50 : 117 :

WAIS Verbal IQ	133
WAIS Performance IQ	117
Difference	16
WAIS Full Scale IQ	127

Dominance, Hand R 9 L 0 Mixed Dom. ____

Dominance, Eye R 10 L 10 Crossed Dom. ✓

Appendix G
Example 3

NEUROPSYCHOLOGICAL KEY

Summary Sheet

Case Name: ____________ Case No. 464

Scorer: JM Date: 6/11/67

TEST	SCORE	
Average Impairment Rating	2.83	0 1 2 (3) 4 5 X
Basic Ratings		
Halstead Categories (total errors)	116	0 1 2 3 (4) 5 X
TPT Time (total) T: 26.0 Bl: 16	—	0 1 2 (3) 4 5 X
TPT Memory	3	0 1 2 (3) 4 5 X
TPT Location	1	0 1 2 (3) 4 5 X
Rhythm	13	0 1 2 (3) 4 5 X
Speech	11	0 1 (2) 3 4 5 X
Tapping (worst hand) (L) R.	42	0 1 (2) 3 4 5 X
Trails B	172	0 1 2 (3) 4 5 X
Digit Symbol	5	0 1 (2) 3 4 5 X
Aphasia	16	0 1 2 (3) 4 5 X
Spatial Relations 4 + BD 2	6	0 1 2 (3) 4 5 X
Perceptual Disorders (total)	50	0 1 2 (3) 4 5 X
Additional Ratings		
Trails A	61	0 1 2 (3) 4 5 X
TPT Time R T: 10.0 Bl: 3	—	0 1 2 3 (4) 5 X
TPT Time L T: 10.0 Bl: 3	—	0 1 2 3 4 (5) X
Tapping R ((Dom.) Non-Dom.)	51	0 (1) 2 3 4 5 X
Tapping L (Dom. (Non-Dom.))	42	0 1 (2) 3 4 5 X
Finger Agnosia R	10	0 1 2 3 4 5 X
Finger Agnosia L	4	0 1 2 3 4 5 X
Finger Tip Writing R	8	0 1 2 3 4 5 X
Finger Tip Writing L	14	0 1 2 3 4 5 X
Tactile Hypesthesia R H (worst): 1 F: —	1	0 1 2 3 4 5 X
Tactile Hypesthesia L H (worst): — F: —	0	0 1 2 3 4 5 X
Suppression Tactile (total) R	4	0 1 2 3 4 5 X
Suppression Tactile (total) L	2	0 1 2 3 4 5 X
Suppression auditory R	0	0 1 2 3 4 5 X
Suppression auditory L	3	0 1 2 3 4 5 X
Suppression visual (total) R	0	0 1 2 3 4 5 X
Suppression visual (total) L	0	0 1 2 3 4 5 X
Homonymous Hemianopia R		0 1 2 3 4 5 X
Homonymous Hemianopia L		0 1 2 3 4 5 X

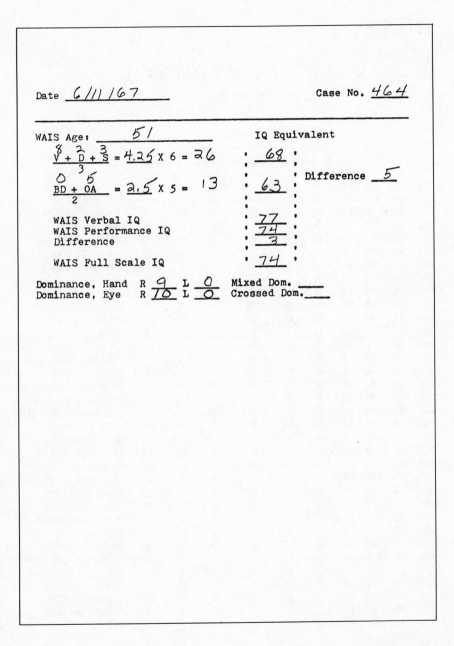

Date 6/11/67 Case No. 464

WAIS Age: 51

$\frac{\overset{8}{V} + \overset{2}{D} + \overset{3}{S}}{3}$ = 4.25 X 6 = 26 : 68 :

$\frac{\overset{0}{BD} + \overset{5}{OA}}{2}$ = 2.5 X 5 = 13 : 63 : Difference 5

	IQ Equivalent
WAIS Verbal IQ	77
WAIS Performance IQ	74
Difference	3
WAIS Full Scale IQ	74

Dominance, Hand R 9 L 0 Mixed Dom. ____
Dominance, Eye R 10 L 0 Crossed Dom. ____

APPENDIX H

Complete Data for All Subjects[*]

No.	Age	IQ	Ed.	Localization Category Key	Psy.	Neuro.	Process Category Key	Psy.	Neuro.	Neurological Diagnosis †
152	29	86	12	D	D	L	S	S	S	Trauma, open head
154	56	127	15	N	N	N	N	N	N	Neg. neurological
157	52	78	14	L	L	L	A	S	S	Abscess, operated
166	49	105	8				S	N	S	Alcoholic CBS
169	30	86	12	L	L	D				Cerebral atrophy
172	45	122	15	N	N	N	N	N	N	Neurosis
176	78	99	16	R	R	R				CVA
180	56	86	16	R	R	R	A	A	A	Tumor, operated
190	75	105	12	R	R	R				CVA
200	57	91	8	L	L	L	A	A	A	CVA
207	73	90	8	R	R	R				CVA
215	42	91	12	R	D	R	S	S	S	Trauma, closed head
218	40	80	4	D	D	R	C	C	S	Alcoholic CBS
228	49	124	16	N	N	N	N	N	N	Convulsive, neg. neuro.
229	43	96	12	L	D	D				Myotonia atropica
235	43	110	13	L	L	D	S	A	S	Multiple sclerosis (MS)
250 ‡	46	98	14	D	D	D	S	S	S	Arteriosclerosis
251	79	101	8	R	D	N				Spinal condition
252	26	100	12	N	N	N	N	N	N	Neg. neurological
253	47	108	12	D	D	N	S	S	N	Spinal condition
255	41	103	9	R	D	D	S	S	S	Huntington's chorea
264	46	93	8	L	L	D	S	A	C	Congenital CBS
265	45	104	7	D	L	N	S	C	N	Spinal condition
267	33	121	20	N	N	N	N	N	N	Neg. neurological
268	47	72	7	L	L	L				CVA
270	41	95	13	D	D	D	S	S	S	Alcoholic CBS
272	39	105	7	D	D	R	S	S	S	Trauma, penetrating
273	56	105	8	D	D	D				MS
276	40	67	9	D	R	R	C	C	S	Cerebral atrophy
280	33	98	12	D	D	D	C	C	C	Congenital CBS
288	52	92	12	L	N	L	S	N	S	Tumor, operated
289	42	107	12	L	N	D				MS

No.	Age	IQ	Ed.	Localization Category Key	Psy.	Neuro.	Process Category Key	Psy.	Neuro.	Neurological Diagnosis †
290	35	106	16	N	N	N	N	N	N	Neurosis
299	34	99	12	N	N	N	N	N	N	Neurosis
301	46	106	18	R	R	D				Trauma, residual
302	46	91	12	D	D	D	S	S	S	Alcoholic CBS
305	68	112	8	L	L	L	S	S	S	CVA
307	43	96	10	D	D	D	C	C	S	Alcoholic CBS
308	48	129	12	N	L	N	N	S	N	Peripheral neuritis
309	68	99	10	L	L	D				Trauma, closed head
324	39	112	16	D	N	L	S	N	S	Trauma, residual
325	50	112	16	N	R	D				Arteriosclerosis
327	49	111	12	R	R	D	S	S	S	MS
331	65	92	9	L	L	D	S	A	S	Arteriosclerosis
337	22	68	12	R	D	D				Toxic, CO
339	49	111	12	D	N	N	S	N	N	Spinal condition
340	77	108	23	L	L	L	S	S	S	CVA
346	62	126	15	N	N	N	N	N	N	Spinal condition
348	43	93	8	N	N	N	N	N	N	Neurosis
356	67	94	14				A	A	A	Tumor, unoperated
357	49	111	12	N	R	N	N	C	N	Spinal condition
359	36	88	12	D	L	L	S	S	S	Cerebral atrophy
363	38	100	10	D	N	N	S	N	N	Neg. neurological
370	42	102	14	N	N	N	N	N	N	Spinal condition
373	55	99	14	D	D	N	S	S	N	Neurosis
376	53	108	13	D	L	D	S	S	S	Alcoholism CBS
380	71	92	8	D	D	D				Arteriosclerosis
381	23	83	13	D	L	L				Trauma, closed head
382	49	94	6	L	L	L				CVA
383	68	90	6	L	L	R	C	C	S	Alcoholism CBS
384	37	84	11	D	D	D	S	S	C	Congenital CBS
386	49	89	12	D	D	D				Alcoholism CBS
393	32	80	12	R	R	D	A	A	C	Congenital CBS
396	41	94	9	D	D	D	C	S	S	Huntington's chorea
400	22	109	12	N	L	L				MS
411	57	93	12	R	R	R	S	S	S	CVA
413	19	94	12	R	R	R				Trauma, penetrating
415	19	119	13	N	D	R				Encephalitis
432	38	106	12	N	R	R	N	C	S	Malformation, operated
434	43	91	12	L	R	D	C	C	C	Congenital CBS
445	43	103	12	R	D	D				MS
449	49	79	5	L	D	D	C	C	C	Congenital CBS
464	51	74	7	D	D	D	C	C	C	Congenital CBS
472	25	76	11	L	D	L	C	C	C	Congenital CBS
486	25	79	12	R	R	R				Trauma, closed head
493	24	87	13	D	D	D				Meningitis
499	48	69	12	R	D	D				Undetermined CBS
502	51	70	9	L	L	L	S	S	S	Trauma, closed head

				Localization Category			Process Category			
No.	**Age**	**IQ**	**Ed.**	**Key**	**Psy.**	**Neuro.**	**Key**	**Psy.**	**Neuro.**	**Neurological Diagnosis †**
506	35	103	10	N	N	N	N	N	N	Neurosis
507	44	77	8	D	R	N	S	S	S	Trauma, residual
513	31	93	16	L	L	L				Undetermined, CBS
516	60	86	8	L	L	L	A	A	A	CVA
518	66	79	8	R	D	D				Cerebral atrophy
524	39	99	7	D	N	N	S	N	N	Spinal condition
526	53	110	11	D	R	D	S	S	S	Alcoholism
560	45	67	12	L	L	L	A	S	A	CVA
562	45	80	8	R	D	L	S	S	S	Undetermined CBS
568	36	133	16	N	N	N				Neg. neurological
571	79	110	13	R	D	L	A	A	A	CVA
593	36	93	12	D	D	D				Trauma, residual
594	26	95	12	N	N	N	N	N	N	Optic atrophy
595	58	79	8	R	D	D	A	S	S	Arteriosclerosis
596	47	81	14	R	R	R	S	S	S	CVA
631 ‡	48	83	14	D	D	D	S	S	A	Undetermined CBS
632	24	107	12	N	N	N	N	N	N	Neg. neurological
637	37	99	12	R	R	D	S	S	S	Alcoholism
638	55	95	7	R	D	D	S	S	S	Alcoholic CBS
640	29	63	12	D	L	L	C	A	A	Trauma, closed head
641	43	92	8	N	N	D				Encephalitis
643	49	108	12	D	N	D				Alcoholic CBS
644	46	75	6	L	L	D				Alcoholic CBS
646	75	89	8	D	D	D	S	S	S	Arteriosclerosis
649	24	94	12	D	D	D	C	C	C	Congenital CBS
651	47	85	8	L	D	D				Undetermined CBS
652	36	99	12	L	L	L				Malformation, operated
656	73	120	21	N	N	N	N	N	N	Convulsive disorder

* Abbreviations:
N = not brain damaged.
R = right hemisphere brain damage.
L = left hemisphere brain damage.
D = diffuse brain damage.
A = acute brain damage.
S = static brain damage.
C = congenital.
CBS = chronic brain syndrome.
CVA = cerebral vascular accident.
MS = multiple sclerosis.
Ed. = education in years.
Psy. = neuropsychological report.
Neuro. = neurological examination report.
Neg. Neuro. = negative neurological, unspecified.

† The diagnoses given in this Appendix were abbreviated from the original neurological diagnoses. Further details concerning these diagnoses are given in Chapter VI and Table 5.

‡ Female.

APPENDIX I

Computer Program for the Localization & Process Keys with Example Printouts

by

Carolyn H. Shelly

Computer Program for the Localization & Process Keys with Example Printouts[1]

```
C               ASSESSMENT OF BRAIN DAMAGE - A KEY APPROACH
C               CAROLYN SHELLY
C FIRST CARD IN DATA DECK INDICATES IF NAME IS TO BE PRINTED
C A BLANK CARD INDICATES THAT THERE WILL BE NO NAME
C A ONE PUNCHED IN COLUMN 1 INDICATES THAT NAME IS TO BE PRINTED
C LAST 4 CARDS IN DATA DECK MUST BE BLANK
C ALL BLANKS WILL BE TREATED AS ZERO SCORES.
C THE DATA FOR EACH SUBJECT MUST BE PLACED ON 4 CONSECUTIVE CARDS.
C THE FORMAT FOR THESE CARDS IS STIPULATED BY THE NEUROPSYCHOLOGY
C  SUMMARY, PROJECT 360, VAH, TOPEKA, KANSAS, REVISED JULY 1968.
C THE FOLLOWING IS THE REQUIRED FORMAT.
C LIST OF VARIABLES READ INTO THE COMPUTER
C VARIABLE                                                   CARD   COLS.
C NONAME = PRINT SUBJECT NAME 0 = NO, 1 = YES                  0      1
C NAME   = NAME OF SUBJECT (0 - 18 ALPHAMERIC CHARACTERS)      1    1-18
C WI     = WAIS INFORMATION SCALED SCORE                       1   20-21
C WC     = WAIS COMPREHENSION SCALED SCORE                     1   23-24
C WA     = WAIS ARITHMETIC SCALED SCORE                        1   26-27
C WS     = WAIS SIMILARITIES SCALED SCORE                      1   29-30
C WSP    = WAIS DIGIT SPAN SCALED SCORE                        1   32-33
C WV     = WAIS VOCABULARY SCALED SCORE                        1   35-36
C WSY    = WAIS DIGIT SYMBOL SCALED SCORE                      1   38-39
C WPC    = WAIS PICTURE COMPLETION SCALED SCORE                1   41-42
C WBD    = WAIS BLOCK DESIGN SCALED SCORE                      1   44-45
C WPA    = WAIS PICTURE ARRANGEMENT SCALED SCORE               1   47-48
C WOA    = WAIS OBJECT ASSEMBLY SCALED SCORE                   1   50-51
C WVIQ   = WAIS VERBAL IQ                                      1   53-55
C WPIQ   = WAIS PERFORMANCE IQ                                 1   57-59
C WTIQ   = WAIS FULL SCALE IQ                                  1   61-63
C PVIQ   = WAIS PRORATED VERBAL IQ                             1   65-67
C PPIQ   = WAIS PRORATED PERFORMANCE IQ                        1   69-71
C IDEN   = SUBJECT NUMBER (ANY 4 ALPHAMERIC CHARACTERS)        1   76-79
C 1                                                            1   80
C WRITE  = HAND USED TO WRITE NAME, RIGHT = 1, LEFT = 0        2    4
C HUSE   = TOTAL NUMBER OF RIGHT HAND USES                     2    8
C EYE    = TOTAL NUMBER OF RIGHT EYE USES                      2   16
C IAGE   = AGE IN YEARS                                        2   53-54
C ISEX   = SEX OF SUBJECT, 1 = MALE, 2 = FEMALE                2   56
C IDEN   = SUBJECT NUMBER (ANY 4 ALPHAMERIC CHARACTERS)        2   76-79
C 2                                                            2   80
C SCAT   = TOTAL NUMBER OF ERRORS ON CATEGORY TEST             3    1- 3
C TPTD   = TIME ON TPT FOR DOMINANT HAND IN MINUTES            3    5- 7
C          ACCURATE TO 1 DECIMAL PLACE, DECIMAL NOT PUNCHED
C TPBD   = NUMBER OF BLOCKS INSERTED WITH DOM. HAND            3    9-10
C TPTN   = TIME ON TPT FOR NON-DOMINANT HAND IN MINUTES        3   12-14
C          ACCURATE TO 1 DECIMAL PLACE, DECIMAL NOT PUNCHED
C TPBN   = NUMBER OF BLOCKS INSERTED WITH NON-DOM. HAND        3   16-17
C TPTT   = TIME ON TPT FOR THREE TRIALS IN MINUTES             3   26-28
C          ACCURATE TO 1 DECIMAL PLACE, DECIMAL NOT PUNCHED
C TPBT   = NUMBER OF BLOCKS INSERTED IN 3 TRIALS               3   30-31
C TPTM   = MEMORY SCORE ON TPT                                 3   33-34
C TPTL   = LOCATION SCORE ON TPT                               3   36-37
C SSP    = TOTAL ERRORS ON SPEECH PERCEPTION TEST              3   39-40
C SRY    = TOTAL ERRORS ON RHYTHM TEST                         3   42-43
C STRB   = TIME TO COMPLETE TRAILS-B, IN SECONDS               3   49-51
C STAPD  =  AVERAGE NUMBER OF FINGER TAPS FOR DOM. HAND        3   56-57
C STAPN  =  AVERAGE NUMBER OF FINGER TAPS FOR NON-DOM. HAND    3   59-60
C IDEN   = SUBJECT NUMBER (ANY 4 ALPHAMERIC CHARACTERS)        3   76-79
C 3                                                            3   80
C VHR    = THRESHOLD ON VON FREY HAIRS FOR RIGHT HAND          4    1
```

[1]Appreciation is expressed to the Computation Center of the University of Kansas for a grant of free time for the development of this program.

```
C VHL    = THRESHOLD ON VON FREY HAIRS FOR LEFT HAND            4    2
C RTACR  = TACTILE DYSFUNCTION RATING FOR RIGHT HAND            4    4
C RTACL  = TACTILE DYSFUNCTION RATING FOR LEFT HAND             4    5
C STACR  = NUMBER OF RIGHT HAND TACTILE SUPPRESSIONS            4    7
C STACL  = NUMBER OF LEFT HAND TACTILE SUPPRESSIONS             4    8
C VFR    = THRESHOLD ON VON FREY HAIRS FOR RIGHT FACE           4   10
C VFL    = THRESHOLD ON VON FREY HAIRS FOR LEFT FACE            4   11
C RFR    = DYSFUNCTION RATING FOR RIGHT FACE                    4   13
C RFL    = DYSFUNCTION RATING FOR LEFT FACE                     4   14
C SFR    = NUMBER OF RIGHT FACE SUPPRESSIONS                    4   16
C SFL    = NUMBER OF LEFT FACE SUPPRESSIONS                     4   17
C RAUDR  = AUDITORY DYSFUNCTION RATING FOR RIGHT                4   19
C RAUDL  = AUDITORY DYSFUNCTION RATING FOR LEFT                 4   20
C SAUDR  = NUMBER OF RIGHT AUDITORY SUPPRESSIONS                4   22
C SAUDL  = NUMBER OF LEFT AUDITORY SUPPRESSIONS                 4   23
C SVISR  = NUMBER OF RIGHT VISUAL SUPPRESSIONS                  4   25-26
C SVISL  = NUMBER OF LEFT VISUAL SUPPRESSIONS                   4   27-28
C FAGR   = NUMBER OF RIGHT FINGER AGNOSIA ERRORS                4   30-31
C FAGL   = NUMBER OF LEFT FINGER AGNOSIA ERRORS                 4   32-33
C FWRR   = NUMBER OF RIGHT FINGER WRITING TEST ERRORS           4   35-36
C FWRL   = NUMBER OF LEFT FINGER WRITING TEST ERRORS            4   37-38
C HHR    = RIGHT HOMONYMOUS HEMIANOPIA, 1 = YES, 0 = NO         4   40
C HHL    = LEFT HOMONYMOUS HEMIANOPIA, 1 = YES, 0 = NO          4   41
C SAPH   = TOTAL ERROR SCORE ON APHASIA SCREENING               4   71-72
C SCROSS = TOTAL SCORE FOR DRAWING TWO CROSSES                  4   74-75
C IDEN   = SUBJECT NUMBER (ANY 4 ALPHAMERIC CHARACTERS)         4   76-79
C 4                                                                 80
C ALPHABETICAL LIST OF VARIABLES
C NAME     VARIABLE                                          SOURCE
C AX     = SUM OF SIGNS STRONGLY LATERALIZING TO THE LEFT    GENERATED
C AY     = SUM OF SIGNS WEAKLY LATERALIZING TO THE LEFT      GENERATED
C BX     = SUM OF SIGNS STRONGLY LATERALIZING TO THE RIGHT   GENERATED
C BY     = SUM OF SIGNS WEAKLY LATERALIZING TO THE RIGHT     GENERATED
C EYE    = TOTAL NUMBER OF RIGHT EYE USES                    DATA INPUT
C FAGL   = NUMBER OF LEFT FINGER AGNOSIA ERRORS              DATA INPUT
C FAGR   = NUMBER OF RIGHT FINGER AGNOSIA ERRORS             DATA INPUT
C FWRL   = NUMBER OF LEFT FINGER WRITING TEST ERRORS         DATA INPUT
C FWRR   = NUMBER OF RIGHT FINGER WRITING TEST ERRORS        DATA INPUT
C HAND   = TOTAL WEIGHTED HAND USES                          GENERATED
C HHL    = LEFT HOMONYMOUS HEMIANOPIA, 1 = YES, 0 = NO       DATA INPUT
C HHR    = RIGHT HOMONYMOUS HEMIANOPIA, 1 = YES, 0 = NO      DATA INPUT
C HUSE   = TOTAL NUMBER OF RIGHT HAND USES                   DATA INPUT
C IAGE   = AGE IN YEARS                                      DATA INPUT
C IDEN   = SUBJECT NUMBER (ANY 4 ALPHAMERIC CHARACTERS)      DATA INPUT
C ISEX   = SEX OF SUBJECT, 1 = MALE, 2 = FEMALE              DATA INPUT
C ISSY   = CONVERTED SCORE FOR DIGIT SYMBOL                  GENERATED
C ITPTL  = CONVERTED SCORE FOR TPT LOCATION RATING           GENERATED
C IWTIQ  = CONVERTED WAIS TOTAL IQ                           GENERATED
C LATE   = DAMAGE LATERALIZED, 1 = YES, 2 = NO               GENERATED
C MDOM   = MIXED DOMINANCE, 1 = YES, 2 = NO                  GENERATED
C NAME   = NAME OF SUBJECT (0 - 18 ALPHAMERIC CHARACTERS)    DATA INPUT
C NONAME = PRINT SUBJECT NAME 0 = NO, 1 = YES                DATA INPUT
C PPIQ   = WAIS PRORATED PERFORMANCE IQ                      DATA INPUT
C PVIQ   = WAIS PRORATED VERBAL IQ                           DATA INPUT
C R      = PERCENT OF IMPAIRED RATINGS                       GENERATED
C RAPH   = RATING FOR APHASIA EXAMINATION                    GENERATED
C RAUDL  = AUDITORY DYSFUNCTION RATING FOR LEFT              DATA INPUT
C RAUDR  = AUDITORY DYSFUNCTION RATING FOR RIGHT             DATA INPUT
C RAVE   = AVERAGE IMPAIRMENT RATING                         GENERATED
C RCAT   = RATING FOR CATEGORY TEST                          GENERATED
```

```
C RFL    = DYSFUNCTION RATING FOR LEFT FACE                DATA INPUT
C RFR    = DYSFUNCTION RATING FOR RIGHT FACE               DATA INPUT
C RPDIS  = RATING FOR PERCEPTUAL DISORDERS EXAMINATION     GENERATED
C RRY    = RATING FOR RHYTHM TEST                          GENERATED
C RSP    = RATING FOR SPEECH PERCEPTION TEST               GENERATED
C RSPA   = RATING FOR SPATIAL RELATIONS EXAMINATION        GENERATED
C RSY    = RATING FOR DIGIT SYMBOL                         GENERATED
C RTACL  = TACTILE DYSFUNCTION RATING FOR LEFT HAND        DATA INPUT
C RTACR  = TACTILE DYSFUNCTION RATING FOR RIGHT HAND       DATA INPUT
C RTAPW  = RATING FOR POORER HAND ON FINGER TAPPING        GENERATED
C RTPL   = RATING FOR LOCATION SCORE ON TPT                GENERATED
C RTPTD  = RATING FOR DOMINANT HAND ON TPT TIME            GENERATED
C RTPTL  = RATING FOR LEFT HAND ON TPT TIME                GENERATED
C RTPTM  = RATING FOR MEMORY SCORE ON TPT                  GENERATED
C RTPTN  = RATING FOR NONDOMINANT HAND ON TPT TIME         GENERATED
C RTPTR  = RATING FOR RIGHT HAND ON TPT TIME               GENERATED
C RTPTT  = RATING FOR TOTAL TIME ON TPT                    GENERATED
C RTRB   = RATING FOR TIME ON TRAILS - B                   GENERATED
C SAPH   = TOTAL ERROR SCORE ON APHASIA SCREENING          DATA INPUT
C SAUDL  = NUMBER OF LEFT AUDITORY SUPPRESSIONS            DATA INPUT
C SAUDR  = NUMBER OF RIGHT AUDITORY SUPPRESSIONS           DATA INPUT
C SCAT   = TOTAL NUMBER OF ERRORS ON CATEGORY TEST         DATA INPUT
C SCROSS = TOTAL SCORE FOR DRAWING TWO CROSSES             DATA INPUT
C SFL    = NUMBER OF LEFT FACE SUPPRESSIONS                DATA INPUT
C SFR    = NUMBER OF RIGHT FACE SUPPRESSIONS               DATA INPUT
C SM     = CONVERTED SCORE FOR TPT MEMORY SCORE            GENERATED
C SPDIS  = SCORE FOR PERCEPTUAL DISORDERS EXAMINATION      GENERATED
C SRY    = TOTAL ERRORS ON RHYTHM TEST                     DATA INPUT
C SSP    = TOTAL ERRORS ON SPEECH PERCEPTION TEST          DATA INPUT
C SSPA   = SPATIAL RELATIONS TOTAL SCORE                   GENERATED
C SSY    = PRORATED SCORE FOR DIGIT SYMBOL                 GENERATED
C STACL  = NUMBER OF LEFT HAND TACTILE SUPPRESSIONS        DATA INPUT
C STACR  = NUMBER OF RIGHT HAND TACTILE SUPPRESSIONS       DATA INPUT
C STAL   = TOTAL TACTILE SUPPRESSIONS ON LEFT              GENERATED
C STAP   = CONVERTED SCORE FOR FINGER TAPPING SPEED        GENERATED
C STAPD  =  AVERAGE NUMBER OF FINGER TAPS FOR DOM. HAND    DATA INPUT
C STAPN  =  AVERAGE NUMBER OF FINGER TAPS FOR NON-DOM. HANDDATA INPUT
C STAR   = TOTAL TACTILE SUPPRESSIONS ON RIGHT             GENERATED
C STRB   = TIME TO COMPLETE TRAILS-B, IN SECONDS           DATA INPUT
C SUML   = WEIGHTED SIGNS LATERALIZING TO THE LEFT         GENERATED
C SUMR   = WEIGHTED SIGNS LATERALIZING TO THE RIGHT        GENERATED
C SVISL  = NUMBER OF LEFT VISUAL SUPPRESSIONS              DATA INPUT
C SVISR  = NUMBER OF RIGHT VISUAL SUPPRESSIONS             DATA INPUT
C TAPL   = AVERAGE NUMBER OF FINGER TAPS FOR LEFT HAND     GENERATED
C TAPR   = AVERAGE NUMBER OF FINGER TAPS FOR RIGHT HAND    GENERATED
C THL    = TOTAL TACTILE DYSFUNCTION RATING FOR LEFT       GENERATED
C THR    = TOTAL TACTILE DYSFUNCTION RATING FOR RIGHT      GENERATED
C TPBD   = NUMBER OF BLOCKS INSERTED WITH DOM. HAND        DATA INPUT
C TPBN   = NUMBER OF BLOCKS INSERTED WITH NON-DOM. HAND    DATA INPUT
C TPBT   = NUMBER OF BLOCKS INSERTED IN 3 TRIALS           DATA INPUT
C TPTD   = TIME ON TPT FOR DOMINANT HAND IN MINUTES,       DATA INPUT
C TPTL   = LOCATION SCORE ON TPT                           DATA INPUT
C TPTM   = MEMORY SCORE ON TPT                             DATA INPUT
C TPTN   = TIME ON TPT FOR NON-DOMINANT HAND IN MINUTES,   DATA INPUT
C TPTT   = TIME ON TPT FOR THREE TRIALS IN MINUTES,        DATA INPUT
C VFL    = THRESHOLD ON VON FREY HAIRS FOR LEFT FACE       DATA INPUT
C VFR    = THRESHOLD ON VON FREY HAIRS FOR RIGHT FACE      DATA INPUT
C VHL    = THRESHOLD ON VON FREY HAIRS FOR LEFT HAND       DATA INPUT
C VHR    = THRESHOLD ON VON FREY HAIRS FOR RIGHT HAND      DATA INPUT
C WA     = WAIS ARITHMETIC SCALED SCORE                    DATA INPUT
```

```
C WBD     = WAIS BLOCK DESIGN SCALED SCORE                      DATA INPUT
C WC      = WAIS COMPREHENSION SCALED SCORE                     DATA INPUT
C WI      = WAIS INFORMATION SCALED SCORE                       DATA INPUT
C WOA     = WAIS OBJECT ASSEMBLY SCALED SCORE                   DATA INPUT
C WPA     = WAIS PICTURE ARRANGEMENT SCALED SCORE               DATA INPUT
C WPC     = WAIS PICTURE COMPLETION SCALED SCORE                DATA INPUT
C WPIQ    = WAIS PERFORMANCE IQ                                 DATA INPUT
C WRITE   = HAND USED TO WRITE NAME, RIGHT = 1, LEFT = 0        DATA INPUT
C WS      = WAIS SIMILARITIES SCALED SCORE                      DATA INPUT
C WSP     = WAIS DIGIT SPAN SCALED SCORE                        DATA INPUT
C WSY     = WAIS DIGIT SYMBOL SCALED SCORE                      DATA INPUT
C WTIQ    = WAIS FULL SCALE IQ                                  DATA INPUT
C WV      = WAIS VOCABULARY SCALED SCORE                        DATA INPUT
C WVIQ    = WAIS VERBAL IQ                                      DATA INPUT
C
      DIMENSION NAME (3)
      READ 25, NONAME
 5    READ 10, (NAME(J),J=1,3),WI,WC,WA,WS,WSP,WV,WSY,WPC,WBD,WPA,WOA,
     1WVIQ,WPIQ,WTIQ,PVIQ,PPIQ,IDEN,WRITE,HUSE,EYE,IAGE,ISEX,SCAT,TPTD,
     2TPBD,TPTN,TPBN,TPTT,TPBT,TPTM,TPTL,SSP,SRY,STRB,STAPD,STAPN,VHR,
     3VHL,RTACR,RTACL,STACR,STACL,VFR,VFL,RFR,RFL,SFR,SFL,RAUDR,RAUDL,
     4SAUDR,SAUDL,SVISR,SVISL,FAGR,FAGL,FWRR,FWRL,HHR,HHL,SAPH,SCROSS
 10   FORMAT (3A6,11F3.0,5F4.0,4X,A4/2(2X,F2.0),6X,F3.0,34X,I3,I2/F3.0,2
     1(F4.1,F3.0),7X,F4.1,5F3.0,4X,F4.0,3X,2F3.0/7(2F1.0,1X),2F1.0,3(1X,
     22F2.0),1X,2F1.0,28X,2F3.0)
 25   FORMAT (I1)
      IF (IAGE .EQ. 0  .AND.  ISEX .EQ. 0) GO TO 20
      PRINT 9000
      IF (NONAME .EQ. 0) GO TO 30
      PRINT 9005, NAME
 30   PRINT 9010
      PRINT 9015
C THE EYE-HAND DOMINANCE KEY
C     SCORE LATERAL DOMINANCE EXAMINATION
C     DETERMINE HAND DOMINANCE
      MDOM = 2
      HAND = WRITE * 2.0 + HUSE
      IF (HAND .GE. 7.0) GO TO 1010
      IF (HAND .LE. 2.0) GO TO 1015
      IF (HAND .GE. 5.0) GO TO 1020
      PRINT 9035
      MDOM = 1
C     DETERMINE EYE DOMINANCE
 1000 IF (EYE .GE. 7.0) GO TO 1025
      IF (EYE .LE. 4.0) GO TO 1030
      PRINT 9050
C     DECIDE IF SUBJECT HAS CROSSED EYE-HAND DOMINANCE
 1005 IF (EYE .GE. 7.0  .AND.  HAND .LE. 2.0  .OR.
     1EYE .LE. 4.0  .AND.  HAND .GE. 7.0) GO TO 1035
C     PRINT EYE-HAND DOMIMANCE
      PRINT 9060
      GO TO 1040
 1010 PRINT 9020
      GO TO 1000
 1015 PRINT 9025
      GO TO 1000
 1020 PRINT 9030
      MDOM = 1
      GO TO 1000
 1025 PRINT 9040
```

```
      GO TO 1005
 1030 PRINT 9045
      GO TO 1005
 1035 PRINT 9055
      MDOM = 1
C     SCORE PERCEPTUAL DISORDERS EXAMINATION
C     ADJUST VON FREY HAIR THRESHOLD TO A DYSFUNCTION RATING
 1040 IF (VHR .GT. RTACR) CALL THRESH (VHR,9.0,7.0,5.0,4.0,RTACR)
      IF (VHL .GT. RTACL) CALL THRESH (VHL,9.0,7.0,5.0,4.0,RTACL)
      IF (VFR .GT.RFR) CALL THRESH (VFR,9.0,7.0,5.0,3.0,RFR)
      IF (VFL .GT. RFL) CALL THRESH (VFL,9.0,7.0,5.0,3.0,RFL)
C     SUM DYSFUNCTION RATINGS FOR HAND AND FACE
      THR = RTACR + RFR
      THL = RTACL + RFL
C     ELIMINATE SUPPRESSIONS IF PRIMARY SENSORY FUNCTION IS IMPAIRED
      IF (RTACR .GE. 3.0) STACR = 0.0
      IF (RTACL .GE. 3.0) STACL = 0.0
      IF (RFR .GE. 3.0) SFR = 0.0
      IF (RFL .GE. 3.0) SFL = 0.0
      IF (RAUDR .GE. 3.0) SAUDR = 0.0
      IF (RAUDL .GE. 3.0) SAUDL = 0.0
C     SUM SUPPRESSIONS FOR HAND AND FACE
      STAR = STACR + SFR
      STAL = STACL + SFL
      SPDIS = (STAR + STAL + SAUDR + SAUDL + SVISR + SVISL) * 1.5
     1+ FAGR + FAGL + FWRR + FWRL
C     PRINT PERCEPTUAL DISORDERS EXAMINATION
      PRINT 9065
      PRINT 9070, STAR, STAL
      PRINT 9075, SAUDR, SAUDL
      PRINT 9080, SVISR, SVISL
      PRINT 9085, FAGR, FAGL
      PRINT 9090, FWRR, FWRL
      IF(HHR .EQ. 1.0) PRINT 9095
      IF (HHL .EQ. 1.0) PRINT 9100
C RATING KEY FOR CONVERTING RAW SCORES TO RATINGS
C     RATING FOR CATEGORY TEST
      CALL SUBROU (SCAT, 132.0, 106.0, 76.0, 53.0, 26.0, RCAT)
C     RATING FOR DOMINANT HAND ON TPT TIME
      RTPTD = 0.0
      IF (TPTD .GE. 10.0  .AND.  TPBD .LE. 1.0) RTPTD = RTPTD + 1.0
      IF (TPTD .GE. 10.0  .AND.  TPBD .LE. 4.0) RTPTD = RTPTD + 1.0
      IF (TPTD .GE. 10.0  .AND.  TPBD .LE. 9.0) RTPTD = RTPTD + 1.0
      IF (TPTD .GE.  8.3) RTPTD = RTPTD + 1.0
      IF (TPTD .GE.  4.8) RTPTD = RTPTD + 1.0
C     RATING FOR NONDOMINANT HAND ON TPT TIME
      RTPTN = 0.0
      IF (TPTN .GE. 10.0  .AND.  TPBN .LE. 5.0) RTPTN = RTPTN + 1.0
      IF (TPTN .GE.  8.9) RTPTN = RTPTN + 1.0
      IF (TPTN .GE.  6.2) RTPTN = RTPTN + 1.0
      IF (TPTN .GE.  4.6) RTPTN = RTPTN + 1.0
      IF (TPTN .GE.  2.7) RTPTN = RTPTN + 1.0
C     IDENTIFY RATINGS FOR RIGHT AND LEFT HAND
      IF (HAND .GE. 5.0) GO TO 2000
      RTPTL = RTPTD
      RTPTR = RTPTN
      TAPL = STAPD
      TAPR = STAPN
      GO TO 2005
 2000 RTPTL = RTPTN
```

```
      RTPTR = RTPTD
      TAPL = STAPN
      TAPR = STAPD
C     RATING FOR TOTAL PERFORMANCE ON TPT TIME
 2005 RTPTT = 0.0
      IF (TPTT .GE. 30.0  .AND.  TPBT .LE. 13.0) RTPTT = RTPTT + 1.0
      IF (TPTT .GE. 30.0) RTPTT = RTPTT + 1.0
      IF (TPTT .GE. 21.1) RTPTT = RTPTT + 1.0
      IF (TPTT .GE. 15.7) RTPTT = RTPTT + 1.0
      IF (TPTT .GE.  9.1) RTPTT = RTPTT + 1.0
C     RATING FOR TPT MEMORY
      SM = 10.0 - TPTM
      CALL SUBROU (SM, 10.0, 9.0, 7.0, 5.0, 2.0, RTPTM)
C     RATING FOR TPT LOCATION
      IF (TPTL .LE. 0.0  .AND.  TPTM .LE. 0.0) GO TO 2010
      IF (TPTL .GE. 7.0) GO TO 2015
      ITPTL = 5.5 - ((TPTL + 3.0) / 2.0)
      RTPL = ITPTL
      GO TO 2020
 2010 RTPL = 5.0
      GO TO 2020
 2015 RTPL = 0.0
C     RATING FOR RHYTHM TEST
 2020 CALL SUBROU (SRY, 19.0, 14.0, 10.0, 6.0, 3.0, RRY)
C     RATING FOR SPEECH PERCEPTION TEST
      CALL SUBROU (SSP, 31.0, 26.0, 15.0, 8.0, 4.0, RSP)
C     RATING FOR TRAILS - B
      CALL SUBROU (STRB, 276.0, 187.0, 124.0, 88.0, 58.0, RTRB)
C     RATING FOR TAPPING SPEED
      IF (STAPD .LE. STAPN + 6.0) GO TO (2025, 2030), ISEX
      GO TO (2035, 2040), ISEX
C     RATING FOR MALE WHO TAPS LESS WELL WITH DOMINANT HAND
 2025 STAP = 100.0 - STAPD
      GO TO 2045
C     RATING FOR FEMALE WHO TAPS LESS WELL WITH DOMINANT HAND
 2030 STAP = 96.0 - STAPD
      GO TO 2045
C     RATING FOR MALE WHO TAPS LESS WELL WITH NON-DOMINANT HAND
 2035 STAP = 94.0 - STAPN
      GO TO 2045
C     RATING FOR FEMALE WHO TAPS LESS WELL WITH NON-DOMINANT HAND
 2040 STAP = 90.0 - STAPN
 2045 CALL SUBROU (STAP, 81.0, 69.0, 58.0, 51.0, 46.0, RTAPW)
C     SCORE SPATIAL RELATIONS EXAMINATION
      SSPA = SCROSS
      IF (WBD .LT. WC  .AND.  WBD .LT. WI  .AND.  WBD .LT. WSP  .AND.
     1WBD .LT. WA  .AND.  WBD .LT. WS  .AND.  WBD .LT. WV  .AND.
     2WBD .LT. WPA  .AND.  WBD .LT. WPC) SSPA = SSPA + 2.0
C     RATING FOR SPATIAL RELATIONS
      CALL SUBROU (SSPA, 10.0, 8.0, 6.0, 4.0, 2.0, RSPA)
C     RATING FOR PERCEPTUAL DISORDERS
      CALL SUBROU (SPDIS, 80.5, 50.5, 30.5, 12.5, 4.5, RPDIS)
C     RATING FOR APHASIA
      CALL SUBROU (SAPH, 41.0, 26.0, 16.0, 7.0, 1.0, RAPH)
C     SCORE DIGIT SYMBOL
      SSY = (WPA + WPC + WBD) / 3.0 - 1.0
      ISSY = (WSY + 3.0) / 2.0
C     RATING FOR DIGIT SYMBOL
      IF (WSY .LT. SSY) GO TO (2050, 2050, 2055, 2060, 2065, 2070,
     12070), ISSY
```

```
      IF (WSY .GE. 12.0) GO TO 2075
      GO TO (2050, 2055, 2060, 2065, 2070, 2070, 2070), ISSY
 2050 RSY = 5.0
      GO TO 2080
 2055 RSY = 4.0
      GO TO 2080
 2060 RSY = 3.0
      GO TO 2080
 2065 RSY = 2.0
      GO TO 2080
 2070 RSY = 1.0
      GO TO 2080
 2075 RSY = 0.0
C     COMPUTE AVERAGE RATING
 2080 RAVE = (RCAT + RTPTT + RTPTM + RTPL + RRY + RTAPW + RTRB +
     1RSY + RSP + RAPH + RSPA + RPDIS) / 12.0
C     COMPUTE PERCENT OF RATINGS IN THE IMPAIRED RANGE
      R = 0.0
      IF (RCAT  .GE. 2.0) R = R + 100.0
      IF (RTPTT .GE. 2.0) R = R + 100.0
      IF (RTPTM .GE. 2.0) R = R + 100.0
      IF (RTPL  .GE. 2.0) R = R + 100.0
      IF (RRY   .GE. 2.0) R = R + 100.0
      IF (RTAPW .GE. 2.0) R = R + 100.0
      IF (RTRB  .GE. 2.0) R = R + 100.0
      IF (RSY   .GE. 2.0) R = R + 100.0
      IF (RSP   .GE. 2.0) R = R + 100.0
      IF (RAPH  .GE. 2.0) R = R + 100.0
      IF (RSPA  .GE. 2.0) R = R + 100.0
      IF (RPDIS .GE. 2.0) R = R + 100.0
      R = R / 12.0
C     PRINT RATINGS AND WAIS SCORES
      PRINT 9105
      PRINT 9110, RCAT, WI
      PRINT 9115, RTPTT, WC
      PRINT 9120, RTPTM, WA
      PRINT 9125, RTPL, WS
      PRINT 9130, RSP, WSP
      PRINT 9135, RRY, WV
      PRINT 9140, RTAPW, WSY
      PRINT 9145, RTRB, WPC
      PRINT 9150, RSY, WBD
      PRINT 9155, RAPH, WPA
      PRINT 9160, RSPA, WOA
      PRINT 9165, RPDIS
      PRINT 9170, RAVE, WVIQ
      PRINT 9175, WPIQ
      PRINT 9180, R, WTIQ
      PRINT 9010
      GO TO (2085, 2090), ISEX
 2085 PRINT 9185, IDEN, IAGE
      GO TO 2095
 2090 PRINT 9190, IDEN, IAGE
C     EVALUATE AND PRINT INTELLIGENCE
 2095 IF (WTIQ .LE. 69.0) GO TO 2100
      IF (WTIQ .GE. 130.0) GO TO 2130
      IWTIQ = WTIQ / 10.0 - 6.0
      GO TO (2105, 2110, 2115, 2115, 2120, 2125), IWTIQ
 2100 PRINT 9195
      GO TO 2135
```

```
 2105 PRINT 9200
      GO TO 2135
 2110 PRINT 9205
      GO TO 2135
 2115 PRINT 9210
      GO TO 2135
 2120 PRINT 9215
      GO TO 2135
 2125 PRINT 9220
      GO TO 2135
 2130 PRINT 9225
C DECIDE IF BRAIN DAMAGE IS PRESENT
 2135 IF (RAVE .GE. 3.51) GO TO 2160
      IF (RAVE .GE. 2.86) GO TO 2155
      IF (RAVE .GE. 2.01) GO TO 2150
      IF (RAVE .GE. 1.36) GO TO 2145
      IF (RAVE .GE. 1.01) GO TO 2140
C     PRINT EVALUATION OF TEST PERFORMANCE
      PRINT 9230
      GO TO 4020
 2140 PRINT 9235
      GO TO 4020
 2145 PRINT 9240
      IF (RAVE .LT. 1.55) GO TO 4020
      GO TO 2165
 2150 PRINT 9245
      GO TO 2165
 2155 PRINT 9250
      GO TO 2165
 2160 PRINT 9255
 2165 PRINT 9265
      PRINT 9270
C THE LOCALIZATION KEY
      AX = 0.0
      AY = 0.0
      BX = 0.0
      BY = 0.0
      LATE = 2
C     DECIDE IF TAPPING SPEED IS VERY SEVERLY IMPAIRED
      IF (TAPR .EQ. 0.0) GO TO 3005
      IF (TAPL .EQ. 0.0) GO TO 3010
      IF (HAND .GE. 5.0) GO TO 3000
C     LATERALIZATION SIGNS FOR LEFT HANDED SUBJECT
      IF (TAPR .LT. TAPL - 20.0) AX = AX + 1.0
      IF (TAPR .LT. TAPL - 10.0) AY = AY + 1.0
      IF (TAPR .GT. TAPL + 5.0) BX = BX + 1.0
      IF (TAPR .GT. TAPL) BY = BY + 1.0
      GO TO 3015
C     LATERALIZATION SIGNS FOR RIGHT HANDED SUBJECT
 3000 IF (TAPR .LT. TAPL - 5.0) AX = AX + 1.0
      IF (TAPR .LT. TAPL) AY = AY + 1.0
      IF (TAPR .GT. TAPL + 20.0) BX = BX + 1.0
      IF (TAPR .GT. TAPL + 10.0) BY = BY + 1.0
      GO TO 3015
 3005 AX = AX + 1.0
      AY = AY + 1.0
      IF (TAPL .GT. 0.0) GO TO 3015
 3010 BX = BX + 1.0
      BY = BY + 1.0
C  POINTS LATERALIZING TO THE LEFT HEMISPHERE
```

```
C      DECIDE IF PERFORMANCE ON APHASIA WORSE THAN ON SPATIAL RELATIONS
 3015 IF (RAPH .GE. RSPA + 3.0) AX = AX + 1.0
      IF (RAPH .GE. RSPA + 1.0) AY = AY + 1.0
C      DECIDE IF TPT-RIGHT HAND PERFORMANCE IS WORSE THAN LEFT
      IF (RTPTR .GE. RTPTL + 2.0) AY = AY + 1.0
C      DECIDE IF GREATER SENSORY FUNCTION IMPAIRMENT ON RIGHT THAN LEFT
      IF (FAGR .GE. 4.0  .AND.  FAGR .GE. FAGL * 2.5  .OR.
     1FWRR .GE. 6.0  .AND.  FWRR .GE. FWRL * 2.5  .OR.
     2THR .GE. 3.0  .AND.  THR .GE. THL * 2.5) AY = AY + 1.0
C      DECIDE IF SUPPRESSIONS ON RIGHT ARE MORE SEVERE THAN ON LEFT
      IF (RAUDR .LT. 3.0  .AND.  RAUDL .LT. 3.0  .AND.  SAUDR .GE. 3.0
     1.AND.  SAUDR .GE. SAUDL * 2.5  .OR.  RTACR .LT. 3.0  .AND.  RTACL
     2.LT. 3.0  .AND.  RFR .LT. 3.0  .AND.  RFL .LT. 3.0  .AND.  STAR
     3.GE. 4.0  .AND.  STAR .GE. STAL * 2.5  .OR.  SVISR .GE. 4.0  .AND.
     4SVISR .GE. SVISL * 2.5) AY = AY + 1.0
C      DECIDE IF RIGHT HOMONYMOUS HEMIANOPIA IS PRESENT
      AY = AY + HHR
C      DECIDE IF MORE VERBAL THAN PERFORMANCE IMPAIRMENT IS FOUND
      IF (PVIQ .LT. PPIQ - 10.0) AY = AY + 1.0
C  POINTS LATERALIZING TO THE RIGHT HEMISPHERE
C      DECIDE IF PERFORMANCE ON SPATIAL RELATIONS WORSE THAN ON APHASIA
      IF (RSPA .GE. RAPH + 3.0) BX = BX + 1.0
      IF (RSPA .GE. RAPH + 1.0) BY = BY + 1.0
C      DECIDE IF TPT-LEFT HAND PERFORMANCE IS WORSE THAN RIGHT
      IF (RTPTL .GE. RTPTR + 2.0) BY = BY + 1.0
C      DECIDE IF GREATER SENSORY FUNCTION IMPAIRMENT ON LEFT THAN RIGHT
      IF (FAGL .GE. 4.0  .AND.  FAGL .GE. FAGR * 2.5  .OR.
     1FWRL .GE. 6.0  .AND.  FWRL .GE. FWRR * 2.5  .OR.
     2THL .GE. 3.0  .AND.  THL .GE. THR * 2.5) BY = BY + 1.0
C      DECIDE IF SUPPRESSIONS ON LEFT ARE MORE SEVERE THAN ON RIGHT
      IF (RAUDL .LT. 3.0  .AND.  RAUDL .LT. 3.0  .AND.  SAUDL .GE. 3.0
     1.AND.  SAUDL .GE. SAUDR * 2.5  .OR.  RTACR .LT. 3.0  .AND.  RTACL
     2.LT. 3.0  .AND.  RFR .LT. 3.0  .AND.  RFL .LT. 3.0  .AND. STAL
     3.GE. 4.0  .AND.  STAL .GE. STAR * 2.5  .OR.  SVISL .GE. 4.0  .AND.
     4SVISL .GE. SVISR * 2.5) BY = BY + 1.0
C      DECIDE IF LEFT HOMONYMOUS HEMIANOPIA IS PRESENT
      BY = BY + HHL
C      DECIDE IF MORE VERBAL THAN PERFORMANCE IMPAIRMENT IS FOUND
      IF (PPIQ .LT. PVIQ - 10.0) BY = BY + 1.0
C      DECIDE DEGREE OF LATERALIZATION
      SUMR = BY + BX * 2.0
      SUML = AY + AX * 2.0
      IF (SUMR .EQ. 0.0) SUMR = 1.0
      IF (SUML .EQ. 0.0) SUML = 1.0
C      EVALUATE THE RATIO OF POINTS LATERALIZING TO THE LEFT AND RIGHT
      IF (SUML / SUMR .GE. 2.0) GO TO 3020
      IF (SUMR / SUML .GE. 2.0) GO TO 3025
      PRINT 9275
      GO TO 4000
C DEGREE OF LATERALIZATION KEY
 3020 IF (AX .GE. 1.0  .OR.  AY .GE. BY + 3.0) GO TO 3030
      PRINT 9285
      GO TO 4000
 3025 IF (BX .GE. 1.0  .OR.  BY .GE. AY + 3.0) GO TO 3035
      PRINT 9295
      GO TO 4000
 3030 PRINT 9280
      LATE = 1
      GO TO 4000
 3035 PRINT 9290
```

```
      LATE = 1
C THE PROCESS KEY
C     DECIDE IF DAMAGE IS ACUTE OR STATIC
 4000 IF (RAVE .GE. 3.0) GO TO (4025, 4030), LATE
C     EVALUATE FOR LOCALIZATION
      GO TO (4035, 4005), LATE
C     DECIDE IF IQ IS LOW AND THERE IS MIXED DOMINANCE
 4005 IF (WTIQ .LE. 98.0) GO TO 4015
C     DECIDE IF IQ IS LOW AND THERE ARE PERCEPTUAL-MOTOR DEFICITS OR
C     IQ IS VERY LOW AND THERE IS A LARGE DIFFERENCE BETWEEN VERBAL AND
C     PERFORMANCE IQ
 4010 IF (WTIQ .LE. 80.0  .AND.  ((RTAPW + RPDIS) / 2.0 .LE. 1.5  .OR.
     1ABS(WVIQ - WPIQ) .LE. 5.0)) GO TO 4040
      GO TO 4035
C     EVALUATE FOR MIXED DOMINANCE
 4015 IF (MDOM .EQ. 1) GO TO 4040
      GO TO 4010
C     PRINT RESULTS OF THE PROCESS KEY
 4020 PRINT 9260
      GO TO 15
 4025 PRINT 9300
      GO TO 4045
 4030 PRINT 9305
      GO TO 4045
 4035 PRINT 9310
      GO TO 4045
 4040 PRINT 9315
 4045 PRINT 9320
C     FORMATS FOR PRINT STATEMENTS
 9000 FORMAT (1H1,76H************************************************
     1***************************)
 9005 FORMAT (27H0NEUROPSYCHOLOGY REPORT ON ,3A6)
 9010 FORMAT (77H0***********************************************
     1**********************)
 9015 FORMAT (30H0LATERAL DOMINANCE EXAMINATION)
 9020 FORMAT (25H SUBJECT IS RIGHT HANDED.)
 9025 FORMAT (24H SUBJECT IS LEFT HANDED.)
 9030 FORMAT (68H SUBJECT HAS MIXED HAND DOMINANCE BUT IS CONSIDERED AS
     1RIGHT HANDED.)
 9035 FORMAT (67H SUBJECT HAS MIXED HAND DOMINANCE BUT IS CONSIDERED AS
     1LEFT HANDED.)
 9040 FORMAT (23H SUBJECT IS RIGHT EYED.)
 9045 FORMAT (22H SUBJECT IS LEFT EYED.)
 9050 FORMAT (33H SUBJECT HAS MIXED EYE DOMINANCE.)
 9055 FORMAT (40H SUBJECT HAS CROSSED EYE-HAND DOMINANCE.)
 9060 FORMAT (50H SUBJECT DOES NOT HAVE CROSSED EYE-HAND DOMINANCE.)
 9065 FORMAT (1H0,32HPERCEPTUAL DISORDERS EXAMINATION,5X,5HRIGHT,3X,4HLE
     1FT)
 9070 FORMAT (1H ,30HNUMBER OF TACTILE SUPPRESSIONS,7X,F3.0,5X,F3.0)
 9075 FORMAT (1H ,31HNUMBER OF AUDITORY SUPPRESSIONS,6X,F3.0,5X,F3.0)
 9080 FORMAT (1H ,29HNUMBER OF VISUAL SUPPRESSIONS,8X,F3.0,5X,F3.0)
 9085 FORMAT (1H ,21HFINGER AGNOSIA ERRORS,16X,F3.0,5X,F3.0)
 9090 FORMAT (1H ,25HFINGER TIP WRITING ERRORS,12X,F3.0,5X,F3.0)
 9095 FORMAT (28H RIGHT HOMONYMOUS HEMIANOPIA)
 9100 FORMAT (27H LEFT HOMONYMOUS HEMIANOPIA)
 9105 FORMAT (1H0,12HNAME OF TEST,10X,6HRATING,8X,27HNAME OF WAIS SUBTES
     1T  SCORE)
 9110 FORMAT (1H ,22HHALSTEAD CATEGORY......,F4.0,10X,21HINFORMATION.....
     1......,F5.0)
 9115 FORMAT (1H ,22HFORM-BOARD, TIME......,F4.0,10X,21HCOMPREHENSION...
```

```
     1......,F5.0)
9120 FORMAT (1H ,22HFORM-BOARD, MEMORY....,F4.0,10X,21HARITHMETIC......
     1......,F5.0)
9125 FORMAT (1H ,22HFORM-BOARD, LOCATION..,F4.0,10X,21HSIMILARITIES....
     1......,F5.0)
9130 FORMAT (1H ,22HSPEECH PERCEPTION......,F4.0,10X,21HDIGIT SPAN......
     1......,F5.0)
9135 FORMAT (1H ,22HRHYTHM...............,F4.0,10X,21HVOCABULARY......
     1......,F5.0)
9140 FORMAT (1H ,22HTAPPING SPEED.........,F4.0,10X,21HDIGIT SYMBOL....
     1......,F5.0)
9145 FORMAT (1H ,22HTRAILS-B..............,F4.0,10X,21HPICTURE COMPLETI
     1ON....,F5.0)
9150 FORMAT (1H ,22HDIGIT SYMBOL..........,F4.0,10X,21HBLOCK DESIGN....
     1......,F5.0)
9155 FORMAT (1H ,22HAPHASIA SCREENING.....,F4.0,10X,21HPICTURE ARRANGEM
     1ENT...,F5.0)
9160 FORMAT (1H ,22HSPATIAL RELATIONS.....,F4.0,10X,21HOBJECT ASSEMBLY.
     1......,F5.0)
9165 FORMAT (1H ,22HPERCEPTUAL DISORDERS..,F4.0)
9170 FORMAT (1H ,16HAVERAGE RATING =,7X,F5.2,8X,18HWAIS VERBAL I.Q. =,6
     1X,F6.0)
9175 FORMAT (1H ,21HPERCENT OF RATINGS IN,15X,24HWAIS PERFORMANCE I.Q.
     1= ,F6.0)
9180 FORMAT (1H ,21HTHE IMPAIRED RANGE = ,F7.2,8X,17HWAIS TOTAL I.Q. =,
     17X,F6.0)
9185 FORMAT (1H0,24HRESEARCH SUBJECT NUMBER ,A4,6H IS A ,I3,15H YEAR OL
     1D MALE,)
9190 FORMAT (1H0,24HRESEARCH SUBJECT NUMBER ,A4,6H IS A ,I3,17H YEAR OL
     1D FEMALE,)
9195 FORMAT (50H WITH DEFECTIVE INTELLIGENCE, AND TEST PERFORMANCE)
9200 FORMAT (51H WITH BORDERLINE INTELLIGENCE, AND TEST PERFORMANCE)
9205 FORMAT (52H WITH DULL NORMAL INTELLIGENCE, AND TEST PERFORMANCE)
9210 FORMAT (48H WITH AVERAGE INTELLIGENCE, AND TEST PERFORMANCE)
9215 FORMAT (54H WITH BRIGHT NORMAL INTELLIGENCE, AND TEST PERFORMANCE)
9220 FORMAT (49H WITH SUPERIOR INTELLIGENCE, AND TEST PERFORMANCE)
9225 FORMAT (54H WITH VERY SUPERIOR INTELLIGENCE, AND TEST PERFORMANCE)
9230 FORMAT (63H THAT FALLS INTO THE SUPERIOR RANGE OF HIGHER MENTAL FU
     1NCTIONS.)
9235 FORMAT (61H THAT FALLS INTO THE NORMAL RANGE OF HIGHER MENTAL FUNC
     1TIONS.)
9240 FORMAT (70H THAT FALLS INTO THE MILDLY IMPAIRED RANGE OF HIGHER ME
     1NTAL FUNCTIONS.)
9245 FORMAT (74H THAT FALLS INTO THE MODERATELY IMPAIRED RANGE OF HIGHE
     1R MENTAL FUNCTIONS.)
9250 FORMAT (72H THAT FALLS INTO THE SEVERELY IMPAIRED RANGE OF HIGHER
     1MENTAL FUNCTIONS.)
9255 FORMAT (77H THAT FALLS INTO THE VERY SEVERELY IMPAIRED RANGE OF HI
     1GHER MENTAL FUNCTIONS.)
9260 FORMAT (77H0THE TEST FINDINGS ARE NOT CONSISTENT WITH THE PRESENCE
     1 OF BRAIN DYSFUNCTION.)
9265 FORMAT (73H0THE TEST FINDINGS ARE CONSISTENT WITH THE PRESENCE OF
     1BRAIN DYSFUNCTION.)
9270 FORMAT (69H0WITH REGARD TO DIFFERENTIAL FUNCTIONING OF THE CEREBRA
     1L HEMISPHERES,)
9275 FORMAT (43H CORTICAL DAMAGE IS DIFFUSE OR GENERALIZED.)
9280 FORMAT (53H CORTICAL DAMAGE IS STRONGLY LATERALIZED TO THE LEFT.)
9285 FORMAT (51H CORTICAL DAMAGE IS WEAKLY LATERALIZED TO THE LEFT.)
9290 FORMAT (54H CORTICAL DAMAGE IS STRONGLY LATERALIZED TO THE RIGHT.)
9295 FORMAT (52H CORTICAL DAMAGE IS WEAKLY LATERALIZED TO THE RIGHT.)
```

```
9300 FORMAT (50H0THE NATURE OF THE DYSFUNCTION IS AN ACUTE LESION.)
9305 FORMAT (58H0THE NATURE OF THE DYSFUNCTION IS A SEVERE, STATIC LESI
   1ON.)
9310 FORMAT (56H0THE NATURE OF THE DYSFUNCTION IS A MILD, STATIC LESION
   1.)
9315 FORMAT (63H0THE NATURE OF THE DYSFUNCTION IS MILD CONGENITAL BRAIN
   1 DAMAGE.)
9320 FORMAT (48H0THANK YOU FOR SUBMITTING THIS INTERESTING CASE.)
15    PRINT 9010
      GO TO 5
20    STOP
      END
C
C            SUBROUTINE FOR OBTAINING RATINGS
      SUBROUTINE SUBROU (SCORE, A, B, C, D, E, RATE)
      RATE = 0.0
      IF (SCORE .GE. A) RATE = RATE + 1.0
      IF (SCORE .GE. B) RATE = RATE + 1.0
      IF (SCORE .GE. C) RATE = RATE + 1.0
      IF (SCORE .GE. D) RATE = RATE + 1.0
      IF (SCORE .GE. E) RATE = RATE + 1.0
      RETURN
      END
C
C            SUBROUTINE FOR ADJUSTING THRESHOLD TO RATING
      SUBROUTINE THRESH (SCORE, A, B, C, D, RATE)
      RATE = 0.0
      IF (SCORE .GE. A) RATE = RATE + 1.0
      IF (SCORE .GE. B) RATE = RATE + 1.0
      IF (SCORE .GE. C) RATE = RATE + 1.0
      IF (SCORE .GE. D) RATE = RATE + 1.0
      RETURN
      END
```

```
*****************************************************************************
                                 Example 1
*****************************************************************************

LATERAL DOMINANCE EXAMINATION
SUBJECT IS RIGHT HANDED.
SUBJECT IS RIGHT EYED.
SUBJECT DOES NOT HAVE CROSSED EYE-HAND DOMINANCE.

PERCEPTUAL DISORDERS EXAMINATION           RIGHT    LEFT
NUMBER OF TACTILE SUPPRESSIONS               6.       6.
NUMBER OF AUDITORY SUPPRESSIONS              0.       0.
NUMBER OF VISUAL SUPPRESSIONS                2.       6.
FINGER AGNOSIA ERRORS                       17.      14.
FINGER TIP WRITING ERRORS                   15.      15.

NAME OF TEST              RATING           NAME OF WAIS SUBTEST  SCORE
HALSTEAD CATEGORY.....      5.             INFORMATION..........  13.
FORM-BOARD, TIME......      5.             COMPREHENSION........  10.
FORM-BOARD, MEMORY....      4.             ARITHMETIC...........   7.
FORM-BOARD, LOCATION..      4.             SIMILARITIES.........   5.
SPEECH PERCEPTION.....      3.             DIGIT SPAN...........  10.
RHYTHM................      4.             VOCABULARY...........  11.
TAPPING SPEED.........      4.             DIGIT SYMBOL.........   0.
TRAILS-B..............      5.             PICTURE COMPLETION...   7.
DIGIT SYMBOL..........      5.             BLOCK DESIGN.........   0.
APHASIA SCREENING.....      1.             PICTURE ARRANGEMENT..   2.
SPATIAL RELATIONS.....      5.             OBJECT ASSEMBLY......   4.
PERCEPTUAL DISORDERS..      5.
AVERAGE RATING =            4.17           WAIS VERBAL I.Q. =           100.
PERCENT OF RATINGS IN                      WAIS PERFORMANCE I.Q. =       68.
THE IMPAIRED RANGE =       91.67           WAIS TOTAL I.Q. =             86.

*****************************************************************************

RESEARCH SUBJECT NUMBER  180 IS A  56 YEAR OLD MALE,
WITH DULL NORMAL INTELLIGENCE, AND TEST PERFORMANCE
THAT FALLS INTO THE VERY SEVERELY IMPAIRED RANGE OF HIGHER MENTAL FUNCTIONS.

THE TEST FINDINGS ARE CONSISTENT WITH THE PRESENCE OF BRAIN DYSFUNCTION.

WITH REGARD TO DIFFERENTIAL FUNCTIONING OF THE CEREBRAL HEMISPHERES,
CORTICAL DAMAGE IS STRONGLY LATERALIZED TO THE RIGHT.

THE NATURE OF THE DYSFUNCTION IS AN ACUTE LESION.

THANK YOU FOR SUBMITTING THIS INTERESTING CASE.

*****************************************************************************
```

```
******************************************************************************
                                 Example 2
******************************************************************************
LATERAL DOMINANCE EXAMINATION
SUBJECT IS RIGHT HANDED.
SUBJECT IS LEFT EYED.
SUBJECT HAS CROSSED EYE-HAND DOMINANCE.

PERCEPTUAL DISORDERS EXAMINATION       RIGHT   LEFT
NUMBER OF TACTILE SUPPRESSIONS           1.      1.
NUMBER OF AUDITORY SUPPRESSIONS          0.      2.
NUMBER OF VISUAL SUPPRESSIONS            0.      5.
FINGER AGNOSIA ERRORS                    0.      0.
FINGER TIP WRITING ERRORS                1.      2.

NAME OF TEST              RATING        NAME OF WAIS SUBTEST   SCORE
HALSTEAD CATEGORY.....      0.          INFORMATION..........    14.
FORM-BOARD, TIME......      1.          COMPREHENSION........    17.
FORM-BOARD, MEMORY....      1.          ARITHMETIC...........    14.
FORM-BOARD, LOCATION..      2.          SIMILARITIES.........    16.
SPEECH PERCEPTION.....      1.          DIGIT SPAN...........    10.
RHYTHM................      1.          VOCABULARY...........    18.
TAPPING SPEED.........      2.          DIGIT SYMBOL.........     7.
TRAILS-B..............      1.          PICTURE COMPLETION...    11.
DIGIT SYMBOL..........      2.          BLOCK DESIGN.........    10.
APHASIA SCREENING.....      1.          PICTURE ARRANGEMENT..    12.
SPATIAL RELATIONS.....      1.          OBJECT ASSEMBLY......    10.
PERCEPTUAL DISORDERS..      2.
AVERAGE RATING =            1.25        WAIS VERBAL I.Q. =          133.
PERCENT OF RATINGS IN                   WAIS PERFORMANCE I.Q. =     117.
THE IMPAIRED RANGE =      33.33         WAIS TOTAL I.Q. =           127.

******************************************************************************

RESEARCH SUBJECT NUMBER  154 IS A  56 YEAR OLD MALE,
WITH SUPERIOR INTELLIGENCE, AND TEST PERFORMANCE
THAT FALLS INTO THE NORMAL RANGE OF HIGHER MENTAL FUNCTIONS.

THE TEST FINDINGS ARE NOT CONSISTENT WITH THE PRESENCE OF BRAIN DYSFUNCTION.

******************************************************************************
```

```
**********************************************************************
                            Example 3
**********************************************************************
LATERAL DOMINANCE EXAMINATION
SUBJECT IS RIGHT HANDED.
SUBJECT IS RIGHT EYED.
SUBJECT DOES NOT HAVE CROSSED EYE-HAND DOMINANCE.

PERCEPTUAL DISORDERS EXAMINATION     RIGHT   LEFT
NUMBER OF TACTILE SUPPRESSIONS        4.      2.
NUMBER OF AUDITORY SUPPRESSIONS       0.      3.
NUMBER OF VISUAL SUPPRESSIONS         0.      0.
FINGER AGNOSIA ERRORS                10.      4.
FINGER TIP WRITING ERRORS             8.     14.

NAME OF TEST           RATING      NAME OF WAIS SUBTEST   SCORE
HALSTEAD CATEGORY.....   4.        INFORMATION.........     7.
FORM-BOARD, TIME......   3.        COMPREHENSION.......     8.
FORM-BOARD, MEMORY....   3.        ARITHMETIC..........     7.
FORM-BOARD, LOCATION..   3.        SIMILARITIES........     3.
SPEECH PERCEPTION.....   2.        DIGIT SPAN..........     2.
RHYTHM................   3.        VOCABULARY..........     8.
TAPPING SPEED.........   2.        DIGIT SYMBOL........     5.
TRAILS-B..............   3.        PICTURE COMPLETION..     5.
DIGIT SYMBOL..........   2.        BLOCK DESIGN........     0.
APHASIA SCREENING.....   3.        PICTURE ARRANGEMENT.     6.
SPATIAL RELATIONS.....   3.        OBJECT ASSEMBLY.....     5.
PERCEPTUAL DISORDERS..   3.
AVERAGE RATING =         2.83      WAIS VERBAL I.Q. =          77.
PERCENT OF RATINGS IN              WAIS PERFORMANCE I.Q. =     74.
THE IMPAIRED RANGE =   100.00      WAIS TOTAL I.Q. =           74.

**********************************************************************

RESEARCH SUBJECT NUMBER  464 IS A  51 YEAR OLD MALE,
WITH BORDERLINE INTELLIGENCE, AND TEST PERFORMANCE
THAT FALLS INTO THE MODERATELY IMPAIRED RANGE OF HIGHER MENTAL FUNCTIONS.

THE TEST FINDINGS ARE CONSISTENT WITH THE PRESENCE OF BRAIN DYSFUNCTION.

WITH REGARD TO DIFFERENTIAL FUNCTIONING OF THE CEREBRAL HEMISPHERES,
CORTICAL DAMAGE IS DIFFUSE OR GENERALIZED.

THE NATURE OF THE DYSFUNCTION IS MILD CONGENITAL BRAIN DAMAGE.

THANK YOU FOR SUBMITTING THIS INTERESTING CASE.

**********************************************************************
```

```
**********************************************************************
                              Example 4
**********************************************************************

LATERAL DOMINANCE EXAMINATION
SUBJECT IS RIGHT HANDED.
SUBJECT IS RIGHT EYED.
SUBJECT DOES NOT HAVE CROSSED EYE-HAND DOMINANCE.

PERCEPTUAL DISORDERS EXAMINATION      RIGHT   LEFT
NUMBER OF TACTILE SUPPRESSIONS         0.      0.
NUMBER OF AUDITORY SUPPRESSIONS        0.      0.
NUMBER OF VISUAL SUPPRESSIONS          0.      0.
FINGER AGNOSIA ERRORS                  0.      1.
FINGER TIP WRITING ERRORS              5.     11.
RIGHT HOMONYMOUS HEMIANOPIA

NAME OF TEST             RATING      NAME OF WAIS SUBTEST  SCORE
HALSTEAD CATEGORY.....    4.         INFORMATION..........   7.
FORM-BOARD, TIME......    3.         COMPREHENSION........   6.
FORM-BOARD, MEMORY....    1.         ARITHMETIC...........   6.
FORM-BOARD, LOCATION..    2.         SIMILARITIES.........   2.
SPEECH PERCEPTION.....    4.         DIGIT SPAN...........   1.
RHYTHM................    4.         VOCABULARY...........   5.
TAPPING SPEED.........    3.         DIGIT SYMBOL.........   4.
TRAILS-B..............    5.         PICTURE COMPLETION...   8.
DIGIT SYMBOL..........    4.         BLOCK DESIGN.........   7.
APHASIA SCREENING.....    3.         PICTURE ARRANGEMENT..   8.
SPATIAL RELATIONS.....    1.         OBJECT ASSEMBLY......   8.
PERCEPTUAL DISORDERS..    2.
AVERAGE RATING =          3.00       WAIS VERBAL I.Q. =          69.
PERCENT OF RATINGS IN                WAIS PERFORMANCE I.Q. =     92.
THE IMPAIRED RANGE =     83.33       WAIS TOTAL I.Q. =           78.

**********************************************************************

RESEARCH SUBJECT NUMBER  157 IS A  52 YEAR OLD MALE,
WITH BORDERLINE INTELLIGENCE, AND TEST PERFORMANCE
THAT FALLS INTO THE SEVERELY IMPAIRED RANGE OF HIGHER MENTAL FUNCTIONS.

THE TEST FINDINGS ARE CONSISTENT WITH THE PRESENCE OF BRAIN DYSFUNCTION.

WITH REGARD TO DIFFERENTIAL FUNCTIONING OF THE CEREBRAL HEMISPHERES,
CORTICAL DAMAGE IS STRONGLY LATERALIZED TO THE LEFT.

THE NATURE OF THE DYSFUNCTION IS AN ACUTE LESION.

THANK YOU FOR SUBMITTING THIS INTERESTING CASE.

**********************************************************************
```

APPENDIX J*

Formal Presentation of the Localization and Process Keys

LOCALIZATION AND DEGREE OF LATERALIZATION KEYS

I. Av. impairment rating < 1.55

NO BRAIN DAMAGE—STOP

II. Av. impairment rating ≥ 1.55

A. Total L b.d. points $\geq 2 \times$ R b.d. points (there must be ≥ 2 L b.d. points)

1. One 2 point L indicator or using one point indicators: L 3 points $>$ R

STRONGLY LATERALIZED LEFT HEMISPHERE BRAIN DAMAGE—STOP

2. Not 1. above

WEAKLY LATERALIZED LEFT HEMISPHERE BRAIN DAMAGE—STOP

B. Total R b.d. points $\geq 2 \times$ L b.d. points (there must be ≥ 2 R b.d. points)

1. One 2 point R indicator or using one point indicators: R 3 points $>$ L

STRONGLY LATERALIZED RIGHT HEMISPHERE BRAIN DAMAGE—STOP

2. Not 1. above

WEAKLY LATERALIZED RIGHT HEMISPHERE BRAIN DAMAGE—STOP

C. Not A or B above

DIFFUSE BRAIN DAMAGE—STOP

Indicators of Left Hemisphere Brain Damage

1. Two Point Indicators

a. Aphasia rating ≥ 3 r.p. more than Spatial Relations rating

(2 points L)

b. Finger Tapping
If R = Dom. R 5 taps < L
If L = Dom. R 20 taps < L
R hand paralyzed

(2 points L)

2. One Point Indicators

a. Aphasia rating ≥ 1 r.p. more than Spatial Relations rating

(1 point L)

b. TPT time R ≥ 2 r.p. L (R or L Dom.)

(1 point L)

c. Finger Tapping
If R = Dom. R < L (in no. of taps)
If L = Dom. R 10 taps < L

(1 point L)

d. Sensory Functions (any one or all of these)
1. Finger Agnosia R ≥ 2.5 × L (no. of errors)
(invalid if < 4 errors on R)
2. Finger Tip Writing R ≥ 2.5 × L (no. of errors)
(invalid if < 6 errors on R)
3. Tactile Hypesthesia R ≥ 2.5 r.p. L
(invalid if R r.p. is < 3)

(any or all of these; 1 point L)

e. Suppression (invalid if there is a loss of primary sensory function in the modality in question rated 3 or 4)
1. Auditory R ≥ 2.5 × L (no. of errors)
(invalid if < 3 errors on R)
2. Tactile R ≥ 2.5 × L (no. of errors)
(invalid if < 4 errors on R)
3. Visual R ≥ 2.5 × L (no. of errors)
(invalid if < 4 errors on R)

(any or all of these; 1 point L)

f. R Homonymous Hemianopia
(Use R & L eye perimeter charts; invalid if total number of functioning squares in both eyes is ≤ 96)
1. R visual field ≤ half number of functioning squares as L visual field.

(1 point L)

g. WAIS $V + D + S$ 10 IQ points ≤ $BD + OA$
$V + D + S = V + D + S \times 2$ converted to an IQ score
$BD + OA = BD + OA \times 2.5$ converted to an IQ score

(1 point L)

Indicators of Right Hemisphere Brain Damage

1. Two Point Indicators

a. Spatial Relations rating ≥ 3 r.p. more than Aphasia rating

(2 points R)

b. Finger Tapping
If R = Dom. R 20 taps > L
If L = Dom. R 5 taps > L
L hand paralyzed

(2 points R)

2. One Point Indicators
a. Spatial Relations rating ⩾ 1 r.p. more than Aphasia rating
(1 point R)
b. TPT time L ⩾ 2 × r.p. R (R or L Dom.)
(1 point R)
c. Finger Tapping
If R = Dom. R 10 taps > L
If L = Dom. R ⩾ L (in no. of taps)
d. Sensory Functions (any one or all of these)
1. Finger Agnosia L ⩾ 2.5 × R (no. of errors)
(invalid if < 4 errors on L)
2. Finger Tip Writing L ⩾ 2.5 × R (no. of errors)
(invalid if < 6 errors on L)
3. Tactile Hypesthesia ⩾ L 2.5 r.p. R
(invalid if L r.p. is < 3)

(any or all of these; 1 point R)

e. Suppression (invalid if there is a loss of primary sensory function in the modality in question rated 3 or 4)
1. Auditory L ⩾ 2.5 × R (no. of errors)
(invalid if ⩽ 3 errors on L)
2. Tactile L ⩾ 2.5 × R (no. of errors)
(invalid if < 4 errors on L)
3. Visual L ⩾ 2.5 × R (no. of errors)
(invalid if < 4 errors on L)

(any or all of these; 1 point R)

f. L Homonymous Hemianopia
(Use R & L perimeter charts; invalid if total number of functioning squares in both eyes is ⩽ 96.)

(1 point L)

g. WAIS *V* + *D* + *S* 10 IQ points *BD* + *OA*
(Computational formulas for *V* + *D* + *S* and *BD* + *OA* may be found in indications of L hemisphere b.d., 2 g above.)

(1 point R)

PROCESS KEY

I. Av. impairment rating < 1.55

NO BRAIN DAMAGE—STOP

II. Av. impairment rating ⩾ 1.55
A. Av. impairment rating < 3.00

1. Degree of Lateralization Key = strongly lateralized b.d.
STATIC BRAIN DAMAGE—STOP
2. Degree of Lateralization Key = diffuse or weakly lateralized b.d.
   a. WAIS FIQ ≥ 99
   STATIC BRAIN DAMAGE—STOP
   b. WAIS FIQ < 99
      x. Mixed dominance present
      CONGENITAL BRAIN DAMAGE—STOP
      y. Crossed dominance present
      CONGENITAL BRAIN DAMAGE—STOP
      z. Proceed to c.
   c. WAIS FIQ ≤ 80 (IF FIQ is 81–98, proceed to r.)
      p. Av. of Tapping and Perceptual Disorders ratings ≤1.50
      CONGENITAL BRAIN DAMAGE—STOP
      q. WAIS VIQ < 6 points different from PIQ
      CONGENITAL BRAIN DAMAGE—STOP
      STATIC BRAIN DAMAGE—STOP
      r. not p or q above

B. Av. impairment rating ≥ 3.00
1. Degree of Lateralization Key = strongly lateralized b.d.
ACUTE BRAIN DAMAGE—STOP
2. Degree of Lateralization Key = diffuse or weakly lateralized b.d.
STATIC BRAIN DAMAGE—STOP

* Abbreviation used:
b.d. = brain damage.
r.p. = rating points.
av. = average.
< = less than or fewer than.
> = greater than or more than.
≤ = equal to and /or less than.
≥ = equal to and /or more than.
Dom. = dominant.
& = and.
× = multiply or times.
R = right.
L = left.
No. = number of.
TPT = Tactual Performance Test.
WAIS = Wechsler Adult Intelligence Scale.
VIQ = Verbal IQ.
PIQ = Performance IQ.
FIQ = Full Scale IQ.
WAIS scales used by the Key:
D = Digit Span.
S = Similarities.
V = Vocabulary.
BD = Block Design.
OA = Object Assembly.

Index

Sid Kriel
244-1761
Ext. 331

17.50 N
G2439
365